YOUR BRAIN ON FOOD

YOUR BRAIN

on

FOOD

HOW CHEMICALS CONTROL YOUR THOUGHTS AND FEELINGS

Second Edition

Gary L. Wenk, Ph.D.
Departments of Psychology and Neuroscience and
Molecular Virology, Immunology and Medical Genetics
The Ohio State University

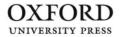

OXFORD
UNIVERSITY PRESS

OXFORD
UNIVERSITY PRESS

Oxford University Press is a department of the University of Oxford.
It furthers the University's objective of excellence in research,
scholarship, and education by publishing worldwide.

Oxford   New York
Auckland   Cape Town   Dar es Salaam   Hong Kong   Karachi
Kuala Lumpur   Madrid   Melbourne   Mexico City   Nairobi
New Delhi   Shanghai   Taipei   Toronto

With offices in
Argentina   Austria   Brazil   Chile   Czech Republic   France   Greece
Guatemala   Hungary   Italy   Japan   Poland   Portugal   Singapore
South Korea   Switzerland   Thailand   Turkey   Ukraine   Vietnam

Oxford is a registered trademark of Oxford University Press
in the UK and certain other countries.

Published in the United States of America by
Oxford University Press
198 Madison Avenue, New York, NY 10016

Library of Congress Cataloging-in-Publication Data
Wenk, Gary Lee, author.
Your brain on food : how chemicals control your thoughts and feelings / Gary L. Wenk.
— Second edition.
p. ; cm.
Includes bibliographical references and index.
ISBN 978–0–19–939327–5
I. Title.
[DNLM: 1. Brain—physiology. 2. Emotions.
3. Neurotransmitter Agents—physiology. WL 300]
RM315
615'.78—dc23
2014014927

1 3 5 7 9 8 6 4 2
Printed in the United States of America
on acid-free paper

for Jane

CONTENTS

PREFACE

Various writers over the past century have compared the human brain to an elegant machine. Imagine that this machine is full of wires and that the wires are different-colored. Some are blue, some are red, some are green, and so on, but they all convey information from one part of the machine to another. Now imagine that the blue wires are organized differently than the red wires, that the red wires are organized differently than the green wires, and so on. If you were to look inside your brain, you would discover that although its pathways are organized like the colored wires in your telephone or computer, it doesn't actually use wires at all but instead uses cells, or neurons, to process information: One neuron is connected to the next and to the next, and so on. Indeed, this elegant machine, your brain, is composed of approximately 100 billion neurons, and within a single structure, the cortex, these neurons make an estimated 0.15 quadrillion connections with each other. These billions of neurons are not uniquely colored, but they do release unique chemicals, called neurotransmitters, onto each other. What happens when molecules of a foreign substance—say, a drug or a morsel of food—interact with the balance of neurotransmitters in this chemical soup? The balance of flavors in this soup will determine what happens to you.

The major point that I want to make in this book is that *anything* you consume—the drugs you take, the foods you eat—can affect how your neurons behave and, subsequently, how you think and feel. In the course of illustrating this point, I examine what neuroscientists currently know about the actions of specific drugs and food in the brain and seek to advance your understanding of your own brain by demonstrating how its workings can be altered by what you "feed" it. So I'll be describing several neurotransmitter systems, including a little about their basic role in the brain, and explore how various substances—be they plant extracts, nuts, mushrooms, spices, chocolate, or medicinal and recreational drugs—can influence these neurotransmitters in terms of their production, their release from the neuron, and their ultimate inactivation and excretion from the body. I also discuss the brain's role in certain experiences—for example, hallucinations, religiosity, pain, and the aging process—and the extent to which these experiences are influenced by what we consume. In addition, I consider the role of evolution in determining the brain's responses to the food and drugs that we consume and place the use of some of these substances in cultural history.

The brain contains over 100 known, or suspected, neurotransmitter chemicals and probably many more that scientists have yet to discover. I have chosen to focus on those neurotransmitter systems most commonly associated with the psychoactive effects of drugs and nutrients that, in many cases, are regularly consumed today.

In essence, this book is intended not as an exhaustive review of all that is known about the topic of food and drugs and the brain but as a brief—and, I hope, enjoyable—introduction to it. By the end of the book, you will know more than just how a select group of drugs or food works in your brain, you will be able to predict how substances that I did not discuss, and those that have not even been discovered yet, might also affect your brain. Even better, you may look back on the chapters you've read and discover that they are much too simplistic for you now and that you want to learn more about greater complexities of brain function than this book covers. If reading this book motivates you to learn more about neuroscience and its associated topics, then I will have succeeded in my goal to advance your understanding of your brain. The suggested readings that I've listed at the end of the book offer an excellent next step in that advancement.

This book could not have been written without the encouragement and generosity of my mentors, colleagues, family, and friends—particularly David Olton, who patiently motivated my curiosity in the effects of drugs on the brain; James McGaugh, who inspired my interest in behavioral pharmacology; Giancarlo Pepeu, who has continued to nurture my interest in the role of drugs in the history of culture; Peabo Bryson, who challenged me to explore the role of neuroscience in religion; Paul Gold, for the many thought-provoking discussions on the Utah slopes; and Jacqueline Crawley, for her boundless enthusiasm and stimulating insights into the function of the brain. Their wisdom helped focus my fanciful ideas into rational theories. I will always be grateful to Catharine Carlin at Oxford University Press for her unflagging support and optimism at the beginning of this long journey. I also feel very privileged to have worked with Marion Osmun and Joan Bossert, my editors, who provided a nurturing combination of advice and encouragement. I am also grateful to the thousands of students who have taken my psychopharmacology classes and whose personal stories enliven these pages. Finally, for more than 30 years, I have been blessed to share my life with a woman of unrivaled intelligence and uncommon patience. Her profound personal wisdom has enriched my life in countless ways. This book is dedicated to Jane.

YOUR BRAIN ON FOOD

CHAPTER I

FOOD, DRUGS, AND YOU

A long time ago, our ancestors discovered that ingesting some plants or the body parts of certain animals produced effects that were rather unpleasant or even lethal. Reference to these substances once appeared in a collection of prayers of comfort for the dying and referred to a type of spiritual medicine, at the time called a *pharmakon*, which was used principally to alleviate suffering near the end of life. Simply put, a pharmakon was a poison. Originally, the term *pharmakos* (φαρμακος) referred to a human scapegoat, who was sacrificed, sometimes literally by poisoning, as a remedy for the illness of another person, usually someone far more important in the local society. Later, around 600 BCE, the term came to refer to substances used to cure the sick. It is, of course, related to two terms in use today: *pharmacology*, the scientific investigation into the mechanisms by which drugs affect the body, and *psychopharmacology,* the study of the effects of drugs upon the brain—effects that in turn are defined as "psychoactive."

This book explores not only several drugs but also a range of foods with these effects. In fact, the single unifying property of these substances is that they are all psychoactive in some way, which means they can affect your brain and therefore your behavior. By the end of the book, I hope that you will appreciate that the distinction between what is considered a drug (i.e., something that your brain wants or needs to function optimally) and food (i.e., something that your body wants or needs to function optimally) is becoming increasingly difficult to define. Indeed, the routine use of some substances, such as stimulants and depressants, is so universal that most of us do not even consider them to be drugs but, rather, actual food. Is coffee, tea, tobacco, alcohol, cocoa, or marijuana a nutrient or a drug? For many people, the distinction has become rather blurred. I suggest that anything you take into your body should be considered a drug, whether it's obviously nutritious or not. As you will see, even molecules that are clearly nutritious, such as chocolate or essential amino acids like lysine and tryptophan (which can be purchased in any grocery store today), exhibit properties that many of us would attribute to a drug.

A SHARED EVOLUTIONARY HISTORY

The foods we eat and many of our most popular psychoactive drugs often come from plants. This fact has led scientists to recognize that the ingredients in these plants are very similar to the neurotransmitters our brains and bodies use to function normally. This is why the contents of our diets can interact with our neurons to influence brain function, and it highlights a very important principle: The food or drug you consume will only act upon your brain if in some way that substance resembles an actual neurotransmitter or if it is able to interact with an essential biochemical process in your brain that influences the production, release, or inactivation of a neurotransmitter. The active ingredients in plants, or their extracts, that we consume are often only slightly modified amino acids or fats that are very similar to the chemicals used by our brains during mental processing.

How is it possible that plants and humans use such similar chemicals for normal, everyday functions? Plants produce chemicals that are capable of affecting our brain because they share an evolutionary history with us on this planet. Even primitive one-celled organisms produce many of the same chemicals that are in our brains. Therefore, whether you choose to eat a bunch of broccoli or a large pile of amoeba, the chemicals they contain may alter how your neurons function and, therefore, how you feel or think.

We have all experienced the consequences of our shared evolutionary history with the plants we eat. For example, unripe bananas contain high levels of the neurotransmitter serotonin. When you eat an unripe banana, its serotonin is free to act upon the serotonin neurons within your intestines. The consequence is likely to be increased activation of the muscles in the wall of your intestines, usually experienced as diarrhea.

Plants are not the only source of chemicals that can act upon your brain. The fact that you share an evolutionary history with insects and reptiles also underlies the ability of venoms, which often also contain serotonin, to produce unpleasant effects you would feel if you were stung by a bee or bitten by a snake. Our shared history with plants and animals on earth leads to some interesting predictions. For example, consider the following science fiction scenario: A spaceman is walking on an earth-like planet and is suddenly bitten by an unfriendly and grizzly looking creature. The spaceman can see that he is injured and that a liquid substance was injected under his skin by the beast. Does he die? No, he does not die, because his species and that of the creature on this foreign planet do not share an evolutionary past or a common ancestor. Although their amino acids might have first evolved in space, as is now believed, since that distant time, their independent evolutionary paths have made it highly improbable that they use similar neurotransmitter molecules within their respective brains and bodies. Thus, every spaceman, from Flash Gordon to Captain Kirk to Luke Skywalker, should feel safe walking around any planet (except their own) with impunity from animal and plant toxins. For this same reason, the intoxicating drinks and powerful medicines that always seem to be popular in these foreign worlds in science fiction movies would also be completely without effect on the brains of our plucky spaceman.

DRUGS AND THE ORGAN OF THE MIND

Back on earth, people in ancient cultures were certainly very aware of the unique properties of certain plants and of the consequences of consuming them on the body and brain; indeed, they often sought them out as remedies for a variety of physical illnesses. This ancient use of plant extracts as medicines was also likely the beginning of a long series of upheavals in our concept of how the brain functions and what its role is as the organ of the mind. For millennia, people believed that mental illness was caused by evil spirits or was a punishment delivered by an angry deity rather than as the result of a brain disease or dysfunction, as we now realize. Only comparatively recently, in the mid-20th century, have effective drugs been introduced for the treatment of mental illness. The realization that it might be possible to treat mental illness in the same way that one treats physical illness—that is, medically—was slow to gain general approval in part because of the wide-ranging, and for some still quite frightening, implications about what this meant regarding the nature of the human mind. What if all mental activity is biochemical in nature? What if our cherished thoughts, such as of God, and our deepest emotions, such as love, are simply the result of biochemical reactions within one of the organs of our body? What does this say about the soul or romance? Will we one day have drugs to treat the broken soul or the broken heart similar to the drugs we use now to treat serious mental illness? It's probably not too farfetched to expect that yes, in the future, drugs will be invented to enhance our romantic urges (Viagra aside) and assist our communication with our deity of choice. Our grandchildren will likely have a whole host of drugs to enhance a broad range of mental functions.

In fact, we already do have a vast pharmacopeia, legal and otherwise, that affect the brain, and no end of debate about their value and effectiveness.

This leads me to several basic principles that apply to any substance you ingest that might affect your brain.

First, these substances should not be viewed as being either "good" or "bad." Drugs and nutrients in your diet are simply chemicals—no more, no less (see Figure 1.1). They have actions within your brain that you either desire or would like to avoid.

Second, every drug has multiple effects. Because your brain and body are so complex and because the chemicals you ingest are free to act in many different areas of your brain and body at the same time, they will often have many different effects—both direct and indirect—on your brain function and behavior.

Third, the effect of a drug or nutrient on your brain always depends on the amount consumed. Varying the dose of any particular drug changes the magnitude and the character of its effects. This principle is called the dose–response effect—that is, in general, greater doses lead to greater effects on your brain, although sometimes greater doses produce completely opposite effects of those with low doses. For example, aspirin reduces body temperature when taken at normal therapeutic doses but increases body temperature when taken at high doses.

Finally, the effects of a drug on your brain are greatly influenced by your genes, the nature of the drug-taking experience, and the expectations you have about the consequences of the experience. For example, if you respond strongly to one drug, you're likely to respond strongly to many drugs, and this trait is likely shared by at least one of your parents.

Sometimes the contribution of your genes to your drug experience can be dangerous. One young man in my class wanted to pledge to a popular fraternity, but he was rather awkward socially and had trouble making friends. He began attending fraternity parties, and against the warnings of his parents, he started drinking alcohol and smoking marijuana. He reported that he became paralyzed after he drank alcohol. It was an odd paralysis that would disappear after a few hours. In the meantime, other students at the party would place his limbs in odd positions, where they remained until the paralysis passed. I asked a physician friend about his condition and learned that the student had probably inherited a disorder of alcohol metabolism. His body converted alcohol into a derivative that was quite toxic to his muscles and so irritating to them that they produced a tightened grip on his body. If he had continued drinking alcohol, then the cellular debris from his degenerating muscles would slowly have collected inside his kidneys, causing them to fail as well. The interaction of his genes and alcohol was going to have devastating effects on his health if he did not quickly change his behavior. There are at least two lessons we can take from this student's nearly disastrous experience. First, get to know your genetic history—you might have some hidden surprises waiting to be uncovered. Second, sometimes, a little basic knowledge about how the things we consume can affect our bodies can actually save our lives.

REALLY BASIC NEUROSCIENCE
AND PHARMACOLOGY

Just how food and drugs affect the brain is the focus of this book, and in subsequent chapters I will provide you with details underlying the specific mechanisms involved in this process. But to ground that discussion, here I present some very basic anatomy and brain chemistry so we can look at the key mechanisms involved in brain–drug interactions.

Why are our brains located in our heads? Wouldn't they be safer if they were deep in our chest, similar to the location of our hearts? Brains, regardless of how small or simple, have evolved at the best possible location to perform their principal function: survival of the individual and the species. With very few exceptions, brains are always located at the front end of an animal's feeding "tube" or mechanism, which in humans and many other organisms is the tubular system (the alimentary canal) that extends from the mouth to the anus. Worms, fish, birds, reptiles, dogs, and you: all simple feeding tubes. Your brain makes it possible for you to find food by sight, sound, and smell and then to organize your behavior so that the front end of your feeding tube can get close enough to taste the food and check it for beneficial or potentially harmful contents before you ingest it. Once the food is in your feeding tube, it is absorbed and becomes available to the cells of your body. Your entire feeding tube and associated organs, also known as the gastrointestinal system, use nearly 70% of the energy you consume just to make the remaining 30% available to the rest of your body. Your brain uses about 25% of the available consumed energy, and your other organs that allow you to reproduce and move around your environment (including your muscles and bones) utilize about 15%. As you can see, very little energy is left over for other tasks in the body. These percentages give you some idea of the priorities—thinking, sex, and mobility—that billions of years of evolution have set for your body to achieve.

THE EVOLUTION OF THE GUT–BRAIN RELATIONSHIP

Brains use a lot of energy, and with the evolution of bigger brains, organisms depended on building longer feeding tubes in order to optimize the extraction of more energy from whatever entered the front end of the feeding tube. For mammals, the length of the gut is significantly correlated with the total body mass as well as with the size of the brain. Over time, as the relative size of the brain became larger as compared to total body size, the forces of evolution changed strategies and developed a more efficient and shorter feeding tube that relies on a high-quality diet (after all, the gut can only be increased in length until there is insufficient room to contain it). Therefore, today modern mammals have a big brain and a gastrointestinal system that is fairly efficient at extracting energy for itself and its principal customers, the reproductive system and the brain. But there was a surprising tradeoff during evolution: As brains became bigger, reproductive success failed. One might predict that having a larger brain would allow greater reproductive success. After all, you would expect that animals with bigger brains would find more food, avoid predators more successfully, and find more mates. This prediction is based on the assumption that bigger brains are smarter, but this is not always the case. Animals with smaller brains and bodies often demonstrate impressive cognitive abilities, while some large-brained species do not. The critical factor is not size but the sophistication of the wiring between individual neurons.

The primate body spends nearly a quarter of its food budget on brain metabolism as compared to only about 5% spent by most other mammals. Our brain uses most of this energy to organize our behavior to socialize with others in our species in order to find a mate with whom to reproduce. That's our inherent biological imperative, regardless of whether or not everyone responds to it. You know one manifestation of this imperative as dating, and it requires a very, very large and complex brain to pull this off successfully. Meanwhile, your brain has evolved some interesting neurotransmitter chemicals that allow you to enjoy dating—two, in particular, are dopamine and an opium-like chemical. Both play a critical role in rewarding your brain—and, therefore, you—for consuming high-calorie food, such as the quintessential dating meal of cheeseburgers and fries at the local diner, and for having sex, often the quintessential dating result. Eating and having sex are obviously excellent ideas if your purpose is to maintain and propagate your species. But these two neurotransmitters, as you'll learn in later chapters, play a larger role in allowing you to experience happiness or euphoria through various behaviors, whether you're eating donuts, having sex, or shooting heroin.

Okay, let's return to the anatomy lesson. At this point, you need only appreciate that your brain is composed of neurons and some supporting cells, called glia. If you were to extract a very small cube of brain tissue (see Figure 1.1b), you would find it densely packed with cells, blood vessels, and very little else. The neurons are organized into columns of cells and small gatherings, called nuclei or ganglia, which tend to be involved in related functions. For example, some ganglia control movement, some control body temperature, and some control your mood.

Overall, your brain is organized so that the back half receives incoming sensory information and then processes and organizes it into your own very personal experience of the here and now. The front half of your brain is responsible for planning and movement, usually in response to some important incoming sensory stimulus, such as someone's voice telling you that it's time for dinner. You hear the voice, smell the aroma of food cooking, feel a craving for food as your blood sugar levels fall, sense that it's late in the day and the sun is setting, and so on; thus, it must be dinnertime. This information is funneled into the front of

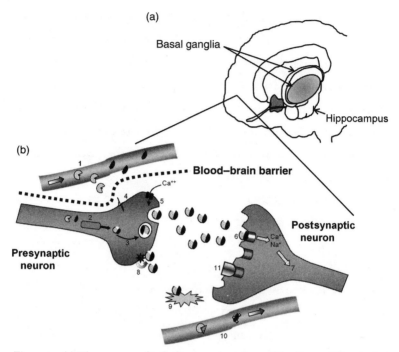

Figure 1.1. (a) The anatomy of a few brain regions that will be discussed later in the book. (b) How individual neurons communicate with each other. See text for details.

your brain, which then makes a decision to move the front end of your feeding tube toward the smell and the voice to obtain a reward—the food and survival for another day!

To facilitate the process between your sensing the external world and deciding how to interact with it and to elicit useful behaviors that will improve your chances of survival, propagate your species, and make you happy, the neurons in your brain must communicate with each other; they do this mostly by releasing neurotransmitters onto each other, including the two neurotransmitters just mentioned as well as others that will be introduced shortly. Most of them can be found in just about every brain structure. Moreover, their function depends entirely on the function of the structures in which they are located.

Let's take a look at a few examples. First, find the basal ganglia in the center of Figure 1.1a. The nuclei that compose the basal ganglia are responsible for allowing normal movement. The level of the neurotransmitter dopamine in these nuclei is much higher than in most surrounding brain regions. Therefore, scientists have concluded that dopamine within the basal ganglia is involved in the control of movement. Furthermore, if we expose your brain to a drug that impairs the function of dopamine or the neurons that produce and release it, then your ability to move will be impaired. But it would be incorrect to assume that dopamine is always involved with movement—it is not. You can also find dopamine in the retina of your eye and in your hypothalamus, structures that have nothing to do with movement. Similarly, the neurotransmitter norepinephrine can be found in the hippocampus, a structure critical for forming new memories. Thus, norepinephrine influences the formation of memories. But norepinephrine also plays a role in other brain regions that have nothing to do with making memories. The take-away point is that there is no such thing as a specifically unique "dopamine function" or an exclusively distinct "norepinephrine function." The brain region that the neurotransmitter is found within defines its function, not the neurotransmitter itself. In fact,

neurotransmitters exhibit a complex array of actions in different brain regions, and so we can rarely make a single universal
statement about their role in brain function.

Neurotransmitters are produced in our brains from the contents of our diets by means of a many-step process. First, *nutrients* (labeled 1 in Figure 1.1b), such as amino acids, sugar, fats,
and peptides (strings of amino acids bound together), are
extracted and absorbed from the food we eat and are transported out of the arterial blood supply to the brain—that is,
they are actively carried through the blood–brain barrier and
transported into the neurons. *Enzymes* (labeled 2) convert these
nutrients into different neurotransmitters. The neurotransmitter molecules are then actively transported into what are called
synaptic vesicles (labeled 3), or very tiny spheres with hollow centers into which about 10,000 molecules of a typical neurotransmitter can be stored for later release from a neuron.

The arrival of an electrical signal (labeled 4) then initiates a
series of further steps. This electrical signal is called an *action
potential*. It is a very small electrical disturbance that moves very
quickly along the axon away from the cell body. The *axon* is a
long, straight extension of the neuron that carries the action
potential and allows one neuron to communicate with other
neurons. Axons are rather like electrical wires that connect the
different parts of the brain. The arrival of the action potential
at the end of the axon induces the entry of calcium ions, which
initiate the next step in the communication of one neuron with
the next: A synaptic vessel merges into its cell wall (imagine two

soap bubbles coming together) and releases (labeled 5) the neurotransmitter into a very small space between neurons, called a *synaptic cleft*. The junction at which two neurons communicate via the release of a neurotransmitter molecule is called a *synapse*. The neurotransmitter molecule briefly interacts or binds with a protein, called a *receptor* (labeled 6), on the surface of the neuron on the other side of the synapse. One consequence of this binding action is that some ions, such as calcium (Ca^{++}) or sodium (Na^{+}), move into the downstream neuron to induce *secondary biochemical processes* (labeled 7), which may have long-term consequences on the neuron's behavior.

Meanwhile, after interacting with the receptor, the actions of the neurotransmitter must be terminated by means of its *reabsorption* (8) back into the neuron that originally released it. This is called reuptake. A secondary method of neurotransmitter inactivation is by *local enzymes* (labeled 9) into a chemical that can no longer interact with your brain. Once the neurotransmitter is enzymatically inactivated, it is removed from the brain into the *bloodstream* (labeled 10). Such byproducts of the ordinary hustle and bustle of the brain can be easily monitored in many of our body fluids, and this information can be used to determine whether our brains are functioning normally.

Drugs and the contents of our diet can interact with any of these various processes and impair, or even sometimes enhance, the production of neurotransmitters, as well as impair their storage into synaptic vesicles, alter their release from neurons, modify their interaction with *receptor proteins* (identified as 11 in Figure 1.1b), slow their reuptake, and possibly even stop their enzymatic inactivation. Because your brain is the organ of the mind, drugs and foods that do any of these things can have a profound influence on how you think, act, and feel.

How do drugs and chemicals in our diet actually affect our brains? Most influence the transmission of chemical signals between neurons. The part of your brain or body where a chemical acts to produce its effect is called its "site of action." The behavioral effects of a chemical can provide clues to its site of action within your brain. For example, nutrients or drugs that affect your sleep or your level of arousal usually alter activity of neurons within a region of your brain that is called the brainstem-activating system. Another clue to a drug's site of action is provided by the unequal distribution of neurotransmitters in the brain. For example, as mentioned earlier, dopamine is highly concentrated in the basal ganglia, a part of the brain that controls movement. Therefore, drugs that affect the dopamine system often impair movement.

Why do some chemicals in our diets affect our brains and how we feel while others have no effect on us? Many drugs or nutrients that might potentially influence brain function are never able to enter the brain because of the presence of a series of barriers; the most important of these is the blood–brain barrier. This barrier allows the easy entry of drugs that are lipid (fat)-soluble and restricts the entry of drugs that are water-soluble. Because the brain is composed of so many lipids, the tendency of a drug to dissolve into lipid and water phases of the brain tells us much about how a drug achieves its effects. Very lipid-soluble drugs enter the brain rapidly; they also tend to exit rather rapidly, which reduces the duration of their action. Some familiar examples of lipid-soluble drugs are the vitamins A, D, E, and K. Nicotine and caffeine are also quite lipid-soluble and enter the brain easily; if they did not, then it is highly unlikely that anyone would be abusing them. Take a moment to appreciate how this fact has been an incredible boon to the evolutionary success of tobacco and coffee plants: Their discovery by our species led to their widespread cultivation and protection as two of the most important plants on earth.

Once a drug has entered the brain, what happens next? Most of the time, the site of action is a receptor protein, which floats on the surface of a neuron. Chemicals that bind to receptors and produce a reaction by the neuron are typically called *agonists*; chemicals that bind to receptors and effectively block the action of a neurotransmitter or agonist are called *antagonists*. Put another way, agonists usually stimulate a response from the neuron, and antagonists usually prevent or reduce the response of neurons. These two terms are used frequently throughout the book.

Some chemicals that you might consume are never completely metabolized or inactivated after they have entered your body and are therefore available to re-enter your brain and continue to affect brain function. In contrast, some chemicals that you ingest are actually metabolized by your body into quite powerful psychoactive drugs. For example, a small percentage of the codeine in cough syrups is converted into morphine, a far more powerful painkiller; psilocybin, from the hallucinogenic mushroom of the same name, is converted into the equally hallucinogenic psilocin; heroin is inactive in your brain and must be converted into morphine before it can produce its euphoric effects. Usually, however, a drug is converted by enzymes to make it inactive in your brain and body and is subsequently excreted in the urine, feces, sweat, breast milk, or expired air from the lungs.

Sometimes the effects of some chemicals are present for so long that the brain slowly adjusts to their presence. Over time, the brain acts as though the drug or nutrient had become a necessary component of normal brain function. You experience your brain's adjustment to the eventual absence of this substance as craving.

CRAVING AND ADDICTION

What does craving feel like? Consider, for example, the very powerful drug sugar. Your brain needs sugar (usually in the form of glucose) to function normally. The many billions of neurons in your brain require a constant supply of glucose to maintain their ability to produce energy and communicate with other neurons. These neurons can only tolerate a deprivation of glucose for a few minutes before they begin to die. Therefore, as blood levels of sugar decrease with the passage of time since your last meal, you begin to experience a craving for food, preferably something sweet. The presence of sugar in your brain is considered normal, and its absence leads to the feeling of craving and the initiation of hunting or foraging behaviors, such as seeking out a vending machine for a Hershey Bar. If you wish to experience the truly overwhelming and powerful nature of drug craving, just stop eating for a full day.

A second, and far less familiar, example of craving would be the response of the brain to long-term exposure to the drug amphetamine. This drug increases the release of the neurotransmitters dopamine, norepinephrine, and serotonin from neurons. The constant presence of these neurotransmitters within the synapse modifies the number and behavior of neuronal protein receptors. Over time, and with daily exposure to amphetamine, the behavior of various neurons may change in profound ways. These compensatory changes partly explain why people who use amphetamine often require greater and greater amounts of the drug to experience a consistent feeling of euphoria. After a few hours, when amphetamine levels in the brain decrease, the individual experiences a lack of euphoria, or dysphoria, which is experienced as depression and a craving for the return of amphetamine back into the brain. The brain, in short, craves chemicals that it "thinks" it needs to function normally; continued craving is called an addiction.

The constant consumption of caffeine, nicotine, or almost any chemical can produce similar types of compensatory changes within your brain and lead to craving with their absence from the brain. This kind of response is exactly what your brain evolved to do for you: Its purpose is to be flexible and learn how to survive, to be plastic or adaptive to a changing environment and to the variety of chemicals that enter your feeding tube. When this situation of "normalcy" is lost because of the absence of something that your brain has become accustomed to having regularly available (e.g., sugar, amphetamine, or anything else that you're accustomed to consuming), your brain reacts by creating in you the urge to replenish its supply. You experience this feeling as craving, regardless of the legality, safety, or cost of the substance being craved.

Craving is also associated with another interesting expression of brain function. The removal of a drug or a chemical from the brain is frequently accompanied by biological and behavioral changes that are opposite those produced by the drug: This is *rebound*. I like to say that the brain always "pushes back." For example, the rebound from the euphoria induced by the stimulants cocaine and amphetamine is the depression that follows once the drugs have left the brain. This interesting brain response is apparently only unidirectional. What I mean by this is that we often observe depression following stimulant-induced euphoria, but we never see euphoria as part of the rebound experience following use of depressants such as alcohol and barbiturates. No one ever experiences happiness as part of a hangover from a night of binge drinking!

Many biological factors such as age and weight play a crucial role in the way that drugs affect the brain and influence behavior. So, too, does the unique neural circuitry that you inherited from your parents and that sometimes influences whether a drug will be exciting or depressing to you. This concept was probably best described as the Law of Initial Value, which states that each person has an initial level of excitation that is determined by his or her genetics, physiology, sickness or health status, drug history, and environmental factors; the degree of response to a psychoactive drug depends on how all of these factors affect one's current level of excitation or melancholy. For example, patients suffering from pain, anxiety, or tension experience euphoria when they are given small doses of morphine. In contrast, a similar dose of morphine given to a happy, pain-free individual often precipitates mild anxiety and fear. If you have a fever, aspirin lowers your body temperature, but aspirin cannot cool your body on a hot day—you must first have the fever for it to work. Coffee produces elation and improves your ability to pay attention if you have been awake for a long period of time or had poor sleep the night before; in contrast, the same dose of coffee is likely to produce much less arousal if you are well-rested. Catatonic patients may respond with a burst of animation and spontaneity to an intravenous injection of barbiturates, whereas most people would simply fall asleep. Sedative drugs create more anxiety in outgoing, athletic people than they do in introverted intellectual types.

The Law of Initial Value is a fascinating concept worthy of additional discussions that are beyond the scope of this book. Indeed, the various basics of neuroscience and pharmacology just summarized barely scratch the surface of all that has been learned over the years about the brain and its response to the food and drugs we consume every day. The chapters that follow build on these basics a bit further to examine the intersection of brain and body chemistry and the co-evolution of our gut and brain within our changing culture. Along the way, we will examine some of the major neurotransmitter systems in detail, including those shown in Figure 1.2.

Almost everything you choose to consume will directly or indirectly affect your brain. Obviously, some things we consume affect us more than others. I'm going to assume that spices, plants, animal parts, drugs of any kind, coffee, tea, nicotine, and chocolate are all just food and define *food* as anything we take into our bodies, whether it's nutritious or not. In order to better understand how food and drugs affect the brain, it will be helpful to divide them into three categories.

First, there are those chemicals we consume in high doses with acute dosing—for example, coffee, sugar, heroin, alcohol, nicotine, marijuana, some spices and a few psychoactive plants and mushrooms. Their effects are almost immediate and depend on how much reaches the brain. In this group, the most important consideration is to get enough of the chemical to its site of action in our brain to actually produce some kind of effect that we can notice and associate with consuming that particular food or drug. Most of the time, this simply does not happen. For example, consider nutmeg: Low doses will be in pies next Thanksgiving, and most of us will not notice that it contains a

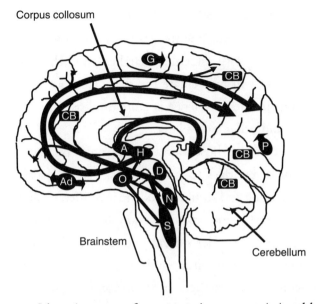

Figure 1.2. Schematic anatomy of neurotransmitter systems. A. Acetylcholine neurons mostly originate within the basal forebrain region and project to the cortex, hippocampus, amygdala, and olfactory bulbs. Ad. Adenosine can be released by virtually every cell in the brain. CB. Cannabinoid neurons are scattered throughout the brain and cerebellum. D. Dopamine neurons originate within the midbrain and project into the basal ganglia and frontal lobes. G. GABA neurons are found throughout the brain as small interneurons and also project from one brain region into another. H. Histamine neurons mostly lie near the bottom of the brain and project diffusely into most brain regions. N. Norepinephrine neurons originate within the locus coeruleus in the floor of the fourth ventricle, under the cerebellum, and project virtually everywhere in the brain. O. Orexin neurons project onto acetylcholine, dopamine, histamine, serotonin, and norepinephrine neurons to promote wakefulness. P. Peptide-containing neurons tend to be diffusely scattered, although there are notable exceptions. S. Serotonin neurons originate with a scattered group of nuclei that lie along the midline of the brainstem and project downward into the spinal cord and upward into all regions of the brain. Glutamate neurons are found everywhere in the brain; they are not represented in the figure.

chemical that our bodies convert into the popular street drug Ecstasy. Yet, if we consume the entire canister of the spice our guts will notice (with a terrible diarrhea), and there is a good chance that we will hallucinate for about 48 hours! According to my students, the experience is quite unpleasant. I will return to nutmeg and other spices later.

Second, there are those foods that affect our brain slowly over a period of a few days to many weeks. This is usually called precursor-loading and would include many different amino acids (tryptophan and lysine are good examples); carbohydrates that have a high glycemic index such as potatoes, bagels, and rice; fava beans; some minerals (iron and magnesium, in particular); lecithin-containing products such as donuts, eggs, and cakes; chocolate; and the water-soluble vitamins. The purpose of these foods is to bias the function of a specific transmitter system, usually to enhance its function in the brain. For example, scientists once thought that drinking a glass of warm milk before bed or eating a large meal of protein made us drowsy because of tryptophan loading. The current evidence does not support this explanation but the claim makes my major point: We must get enough of any particular nutrient or chemical to the right place and at the right dose in our brain in order for us to notice any effects. Unfortunately, tryptophan has difficulty getting into our brain, particularly when consumed within the context of a large variety of other amino acids, as are present in meat.

So, what is the scientific evidence for considering the cognitive effects of these foods? Mostly, it's related to what happens when we do not get enough of them. For example, studies have shown that consuming too little tryptophan makes us depressed and angry; historians now blame low-tryptophan diets for multiple wars and acts of cannibalism. Too little of water-soluble vitamins (the B's and C) in the diet will induce changes in brain function that we will begin to notice after a few weeks of deprivation. Many authors naively jump to the conclusion that giving high doses of such nutrients will rapidly improve our mood or thinking. Sadly, this is rarely the case. Ordinarily, the foods in this category require more time to affect our brains than do those foods in the first category.

The third category includes the slow-acting, lifetime dosing nutrients that are always in the popular press. This category includes the antioxidant-rich foods such as colorful fruit and vegetables, fish and olive oils, fruit juices, anti-inflammatory plants and drugs such as aspirin, some steroids, cinnamon and some other spices, nicotine, caffeine and chocolate, the fat-soluble vitamins, nuts, legumes, beer, and red wine. People who eat these foods positively benefit from consuming them regularly over their life span. The benefit comes from the fact that all of these foods provide our brains with some form of protection against the most deadly thing we expose ourselves to every day—oxygen. Because we consume food, we must consume oxygen. Because we consume oxygen, we age. Thus, people who live the longest tend to eat foods rich in antioxidants or simply eat much less food. Although nicotine and caffeine prevent the toxic actions of oxygen in our brain, I am not suggesting that anyone should smoke with their morning coffee.

You can see that, depending on how you frame the question about how food affects the brain, you get a different list of foods and a different reason for consuming them. If you wish to alter your current brain function or slow your brain's aging, you need to eat specific foods. In truth, no one ever considers these distinctions when eating—we just eat what tastes good. Sadly, our brains powerfully reward us when we eat sugar, fat, and salt; thus we have obesity and the oncoming epidemic of obesity-related illnesses. Consequently, like drugs, food has both negative and positive effects, and it all depends on what drug or food you take, how much you consume, and for how long. In later sections I'll discuss the neurological mechanisms that control our urge to keep eating tasty foods.

CHAPTER 2

NEUROBIOLOGY OF FEEDING: HORMONES, OVEREATING, AND AGING

The brain receives a steady stream of varied hormonal signals about the stored energy status of the body. After careful consideration of environmental factors, such as when another food source might next be available, consideration of anticipated energy needs during that time period, and the current social situation, the brain attempts to influence food choices according to how nutritional it is, how pleasurable it tastes, and past experience with the source—and then eating begins. But the real challenge for the brain is how to stop eating.

This decision is partly determined by how fat we are. The brain learns about this through the action of two hormones—leptin and insulin—and responds by reducing food consumption. The blood levels of insulin and leptin are continuously elevated in the brains of obese people, but their brains ignore these hormonal signals and so eating continues. The effectiveness of these hormones is influenced by fluctuating levels of estrogen; this leads to the gender dichotomy that females are more sensitive to the appetite-suppressant action of leptin (initiated by their body fat), whereas males are sensitive to the appetite-suppressant action of insulin (induced by eating). Female brains on food do not follow the same rules as male brains on food.

The brain also gets sensory feedback from the mouth and nose about the smell, taste, and feel of the food, as well as the expansion of the stomach. Unfortunately, these signals can easily be ignored by the brain—and so we keep eating. New research on how the brain gets us to stop eating has led to the development of drugs designed to reduce food intake by mimicking one or more of these feedback signals. But each time the same thing happens—caloric intake decreases for a short time and then the brain learns to ignore the false signal so that caloric intake is restored. Why? Because the consequences of not ingesting a sufficient number of calories has dire consequences for our survival. There is no evolutionary advantage to trying to lose weight by restricting eating. Four billion years of evolution have led to the following simple directive: Find and consume the energy within food, repeat often. Think about this next time you contemplate taking a diet aid.

When an energy source is on the tongue, the brain is informed via six quite simple molecular interactions within the taste buds that lead to the activation of reward pathways in the brain that utilize the neurotransmitters dopamine, endorphins, endocannabinoids, and orexin. Orexin influences both our level of arousal and our craving for food. Take a moment to appreciate how this system optimizes your daily existence and survival. These orexin neurons wake you in the morning and then make you crave food.

Once food reaches the gut it encounters still more receptors that detect sweetness, fattiness, and bitterness. It appears as though the entire gut is a continuation of the tongue with specialized taste receptors. The activation of these receptors slows the intestinal transit of the food, providing a greater opportunity for nutrient extraction within the limited length of the intestines.

BIORYHTHMS AND DIET EFFECTS ON THE BRAIN

Is there a good time of day to eat? What would happen if you could only eat between the hours of 9 am and 4 pm? Would you gain less weight and be healthier overall even if you ate a high-fat diet? The answer is yes and is based on how the body is influenced by our daily rhythms of eating and sleeping. We are already well aware of the negative consequences of ignoring the role of our biorhythms: Nightshift work, and the odd patterns of sleeping and waking that this lifestyle involves, has many negative health consequences, including insomnia, high blood pressure, obesity, high triglyceride levels, and diabetes—collectively known as the metabolic syndrome.

In a recent study mice were given free access to a nutrition-
ally balanced diet or a diet that was high (61% of calories!) in
fat. Some mice were allowed total access to the food at all times;
others were only allowed access for an 8-hour window during
the early phase of their normal active period. Mice given total
all-day access to a high-fat diet (the standard American diet)
developed obesity, diabetes, and metabolic syndrome and poor
sleep–wake rhythms. Now for the good news! The mice that
had time-restricted access to the high-fat diet were significantly
healthier than the mice given all-day access to the same diet.
These lucky mice lost body fat and had normal glucose tolerance, reduced serum cholesterol, improved motor function, and
normal sleep cycles. Most surprising, the daily caloric intake of
all groups did not differ, regardless of their diet or feeding
schedule. Therefore, it truly does matter when you eat. The
take-home message is eat early, skip dinner, and never have
late-night snacks. Skipping breakfast and then overeating in the
evening play a significant role in weight gain and obesity.
Furthermore, people who skip breakfast report not feeling as
satisfied by their food and being hungry between meals. If this
sounds like you, then it's time to change your mealtimes.

WHEN GOOD FOOD TURNS BAD

Our body's reaction to the food we eat can sometimes warn us
that something is wrong. One day we're eating our favorite food
without consequence; the next day, the same food produces
nausea, dizziness, and mental confusion. Why? Sometimes the

constituents of our diet can induce toxic reactions when they are not being properly metabolized and excreted. For example, starfruit (*Averrhoa carambola*)—small, waxy-skinned fruit whose name originated from the star-like shape produced when the fruit is cut in cross section—contain an impressive variety of vitamins, minerals, and dietary fibers and are a rich source of antioxidants. But they pose a serious risk for individuals with kidney failure. The consequences of eating starfruit when the kidneys are not functioning adequately include several symptoms that might easily be ignored or misinterpreted as unrelated to eating the fruit, such as vomiting, hiccups, mental confusion, and seizures. Overall, this is a very important warning: How we respond to the components of our diet is greatly influenced by the status of our health.

ACIDIC DIETS AND BRAIN FUNCTION

Is it true that the foods and beverages you consume can cause your blood to become more alkaline or acidic? Contrary to popular hype, the answer is no, not to any significant degree. The pH of your blood is tightly regulated by a complex system of buffers that are continuously at work to maintain a normal level that is slightly more alkaline than pure water. The bottom line is that if you're breathing and going about your daily activities, your body is doing an adequate job of keeping your blood pH under control and your diet is not causing any wild deviations of your blood pH.

Your blood (plasma) needs to maintain a pH of 7.35 to 7.45 for your cells to function properly. While the various reasons your cells require your blood to maintain a pH in this range to stay healthy are beyond the scope of this book, it is worth mentioning the most important reason: All of the proteins that work in your body have to maintain a specific geometric shape in order to function, and the three-dimensional shapes of the proteins in your body are affected by the tiniest changes in the pH of your body fluids.

When people encourage you to "alkalize your blood," they mean that you should eat plenty of foods that have an alkaline-forming effect on your entire body. The reason is that the vast majority of highly processed foods—such as white flour products and sugar—have an acid-forming effect on your system, and if you spend years eating a poor diet that is mainly acid-forming, you will overwork some of the buffering systems to a point where you could create undesirable changes in your health. Generally speaking, most vegetables and fruits have an alkaline-forming effect on your body, while most grains, animal foods, and highly processed foods have an acid-forming effect. Your health is best served by a mixture of nutrient-dense, alkaline- and acid-forming foods that include carbohydrates, fats, and proteins. Let's take a look at these foods.

CARBOHYDRATES AND BRAIN FUNCTION

A *carbohydrate* is a molecule made of carbon, hydrogen, and oxygen. Glucose is a carbohydrate and is commonly called "sugar." The adult brain has a very high energy demand requiring continuous delivery of glucose from blood. The brain accounts for approximately 2% of the body weight but consumes approximately 20% of glucose-derived energy, making it the main consumer of glucose. The largest proportion of energy in the brain is consumed for neuronal computation and information processing.

Obviously, our brain needs a lot of sugar; without it we quickly lose the ability to think and slip into a coma. We must obtain the sugar from our diet. Sadly, somewhere in our evolutionary history, we lost the ability to convert fat into sugar; unlike a few lucky animals, humans cannot perform this metabolic trick. So, in the morning when you wake up from a long period of fasting, your brain wants you to eat lots of sugar and other simple carbohydrate sources, such as a donut. There is a reason that donuts and sugar-laden cereals are so popular, and you can lay the blame on neurons within the feeding center of your hypothalamus. This mechanism works nicely. First thing in the morning you eat lots of simple, easily digestible sugars and your brain rewards you with a good feeling by releasing dopamine and endogenous opiates. Your brain needs the sugar to produce chemicals that are critical for learning and memory. Impaired glucose regulation correlates with impaired learning in the elderly and leads to Alzheimer's disease. Scientists have recently discovered that the inability of specific brain regions to efficiently use glucose precedes the degeneration of those same brain region decades later. Sadly, eating more sugar is not the answer to preventing dementia. Indeed, consuming large amounts of sugar is not healthy for your pancreas or cardiovascular system. What's good for the brain is not always good for the other organs of your body.

GOOD FAT AND BAD FAT

We need fat. Fat frequently takes up more territory than any other organ in our bodies. A long time ago, our ancestors needed fat deposits because food was not always available. Fat can accommodate wide swings in nutrient availability because it is capable of rapid changes in size, especially our subcutaneous fat, which is not subject to size constraints. We can simply keep packing on the fat cells for a future time when less food might be available—thus improving our chances of survival.

In humans, fat is purposefully located beneath the skin and around our vital organs, where it can protect our body against infection and trauma. Bacterial and fungal infections of fat are uncommon and cancer metastases into fat pads are rare; this is likely related to the high local concentrations of fatty acid that are lethal to pathogens and non-fat cells. Fat is also critical for thermoregulation, by preventing heat loss and acting as insulation and by generating heat in brown fat—a specialized fat deposit that lies between the shoulder blades and is rich in mitochondria. Fat provides physical protection and forms a buffer that dissipates pressure over skeletal prominences such as elbows and knees, thus preventing the skin from collapsing at vulnerable spots on our limbs.

Our fat mass increases throughout middle age; then, it starts being redistributed. It moves from subcutaneous deposits to visceral deposits around our vital organs. Given this redistribution, waist size tends to increase. To make matters worse, as we age our fat is also being redistributed into bone marrow, muscle, and liver. This loss of subcutaneous fat is often associated with the development of metabolic syndrome, characterized by glucose intolerance, insulin resistance, visceral obesity, and hypertension. When present in the elderly, this condition impairs cardiovascular function and accelerates cognitive decline. Some of us inherit a tendency to redistribute our fat at an earlier age, and at a faster rate; when this happens, it is associated with a reduced life span.

Sadly, standard liposuction is not going to help. Removing large amounts of subcutaneous fat does not improve insulin sensitivity. Indeed, having larger amounts of subcutaneous fat might actually be protective if you are obese. In contrast to the removal of subcutaneous fat by liposuction, the removal of visceral fat—the fat that forms around the organ inside the body, actually enhances insulin sensitivity and extends maximum life span. The reason for this is that all fat deposits do not behave similarly; visceral fat is more proinflammatory than subcutaneous fat. Obesity and aging are both associated with chronic, low-grade, body-wide inflammation and insulin resistance. Fat dysfunction associated with obesity is now thought to reproduce many of the same metabolic conditions that underlie the normal aging process. Essentially, obesity accelerates the aging of our organs and predisposes us to diseases that are common in old age. But you do not have to be obese in order to suffer from the consequences of excess fat cells. Even skinny older people with relatively more visceral fat than subcutaneous fat are at increased risk for mortality.

Because surgical removal of visceral fat is not an easy option, the only solution available is to eat less food. Caloric restriction is the only valid, scientifically proven dietary intervention that has been shown to slow the aging process and improve overall health. The reason we hear so little about this approach is because no one stands to make a profit on all of us eating less food.

Dietary Fats That Improve Brain Function

We have a fatty brain, and fat plays many vital roles in brain function. In the past, very little attention was given to the influence of dietary fats on our mental state. Recent evidence indicates that it might be possible to manipulate our dietary fat intake to treat or prevent disorders of cognitive function.

A recent study compared the effects of monounsaturated fats from olive and canola oils with polyunsaturated fats from meat, fish, and vegetable oils on a variety of biochemical changes and electrical properties of cells within a brain region that is critical for learning and memory. After 11 months, a diet high in monounsaturated fats, often referred to as the Mediterranean diet, altered brain chemistry in such a way that learning was enhanced, age-related cognitive decline slowed, and the risk of getting Alzheimer's disease was reduced. These findings support the addition of canola, olive, and fish oils to our diet and further demonstrate that sensible nutritional choices are vital for optimal brain function and good mental health.

Omega-3s

Omega-3 fatty acids are a family of fats that occur naturally; three of them, α-linolenic acid (ALA), eicosapentaenoic acid, and docosahexaenoic acid (DHA), are important components of the human diet. Some recent studies have concluded that being deficient in omega-3 fatty acids may affect brain physiology and increase the risk of cognitive decline. Superficially, this claim makes sense. After all, DHA is abundant in the brain and is involved in numerous critical functions. It may also enhance learning and memory processes in the brain.

Dietary intake of omega-3s, mainly from fish, have been claimed to slow cognitive decline and the incidence of dementia. The problem is that thus far all of the clinical trials have either included too few patients or were conducted for quite brief periods of time. Thus, the results tended to be rather variable and potentially misleading. Recently, a study investigating the potential benefit of omega-3s followed almost 3,000 people, aged 60 to 80 years, for 40 months. Their daily diets, medications, and health status were carefully monitored. The patients and their controls were carefully matched for education level, smoking habits, and alcohol use, among other features. Simply stated, omega-3 intake (as fish or pill supplement) provided no benefits. Cognitive decline was unaffected. What does this mean? A single, good dietary habit is not enough to provide protection for your aging brain.

In contrast to their lack of benefit for age-related cognitive decline, omega-3 fatty acids may have a beneficial influence on the outcome in depressive disorders. Chronic diet supplementation with omega-3 fatty acids has produced antidepressant-like effects similar to those with common antidepressant drugs. The therapeutic approach of combining omega-3 fatty acids with low doses of antidepressants might represent benefits in the treatment of depression, especially in patients with depression resistant to conventional treatments or by decreasing the magnitude of some antidepressant dose-dependent side effects.

Bad Fat and Brain Function

We know that obesity is associated with hypertension, diabetes, sleep apnea, and numerous arthritic disorders. Unfortunately, obese individuals also perform worse in neurocognitive tests even when controlled for education level and evidence of depression. Furthermore, women who eat an unhealthy high-fat diet prior to and during pregnancy are more likely to give birth to children, particularly males, who are at risk of abnormal behaviors, predominantly anxiety, during adulthood. Physicians frequently warn pregnant women to monitor their caloric intake and maintain a healthy weight before and during pregnancy. Maternal nutritional status, infection, and physical or psychological trauma during pregnancy can all increase the risk of obesity, diabetes, and mental disorders in offspring. In the past, the concern was maternal malnutrition—that is, the developing fetus might lack critical nutrients for normal growth. Today, in the United States, the concern has shifted to overnutrition and obesity and the risks faced by the developing fetal brain.

Another study of maternal obesity reported serious inattention problems and a two-fold increase in the incidence of impaired emotional regulation that was still evident 5 years after birth. Maternal obesity also causes abnormalities in areas of the brain responsible for feeding behavior and memory. All of these changes were most noticeable in male offspring. How does maternal obesity impair fetal brain development? Once again, the damage is due to the fact that fat cells release inflammatory proteins, called cytokines, into the body and brain. The more fat cells the mother has, the more cytokines get released into her blood.

Obesity also increases the likelihood of becoming depressed. Depression is often referred to as "the common cold of mental illness." This reference reveals some fundamental insights into why we become depressed when we are suffering with the flu or a bacterial infection. Bacteria induce our bodies to release cytokines; depressive behaviors are now thought to be caused by elevated levels of cytokines in the brain. The additional inflammation may also explain why many antidepressant drugs are less effective in obese or elderly people: Their brains have elevated levels of cytokines. Exercise can modestly reduce the level of cytokines in the brain and depressed obese people often find some relief by exercising. Overall, staying thin means you'll be less depressed and live longer.

THE PLEASURE OF OVEREATING

Two different neurotransmitter systems, endogenous opioid peptides called *endorphins* and *cannabinoids*, make eating pleasurable. Endorphins enhance the sensory pleasure derived from food, and the consumption of foods high in fat and sugar stimulates the release of endorphins. Endorphins enable us to experience the deliciousness of food and ensure that we do not stop eating too soon, but they don't influence our decision to eat. Drugs that selectively block the action of endorphins reduce the intake of foods that are quite sweet or have a high fat content. Interestingly, these drugs that block endorphins, called antagonists, only reduce the pleasure of eating these foods; they do not reduce the feelings of hunger. Endorphins drive us to overconsume palatable foods by blunting the impact of feeling full. As we all know, while standing next to the buffet table, we will engage in mindless eating. We know that we should stop eating and move away from the buffet line and let someone else get at the food. Our bellies are full to the point that it hurts to breathe. Belts are loosened another notch. Why can't we stop eating?

Neuroscientists have some interesting explanations. One of these is called "ingestion analgesia" and it involves endorphins. The role of ingestion analgesia is to keep you eating. Even though continued eating has become unpleasant because the stomach is painfully stretched to its full capacity and we've reached the point where we cannot unbutton anything else in public, and even though we've embarrassed ourselves in front of the relatives or coworkers by our voracious appetite, we still keep noshing. Essentially, we block out the painful feedback from these feelings by releasing endogenous opiates into our brain and body. Not surprising, our reaction to pain is significantly reduced when eating tasty foods, such as chocolate. This explains why we can indulge in a decadent dessert even after we've become fully satiated by a large meal. We have basically become insensitive to the pain of continued eating.

Our brains evolved when food was scarce; thus, we are compelled by our genetic legacy to eat whatever and whenever possible. Animals have a tendency to eat a great deal of food when palatable food is readily available. Not only that, but we also subconsciously prevent others from taking our food source. We defend our access to tasty food when it is within easy reach and is at risk of being consumed by other humans. Studies have shown that humans will eat more when more food is available even when the food is stale or otherwise unappealing (which is good news for bad cooks!). Furthermore, even if you point out to someone that the food is stale or that they've eaten more than their fair share, they will continue to eat. Our biological drive to consume tasty foods to completion outweighs any opposing cognitive or motivational factors. Even after we've gained a lot of weight, our bodies want to gain more.

Research indicates that obese humans have elevated levels of endogenous endocannabinoids—marijuana-like chemicals—in the blood and brain. Remember the munchies? When we become overweight our bodies induce a constant state of the munchies by bathing our brain in endocannabinoids.

The endogenous marijuana neurotransmitters, the endocannabinoids, also contribute to the pleasurable aspect of eating. Scientists have discovered that marijuana increased the pleasurable response to eating sugar but had no effect on how much we dislike the taste of other types of foods. For example, if you hate eating peas or broccoli, smoking marijuana will not induce you to like eating them. The ability of sugar to induce a rewarding feeling is caused by the release of dopamine in the brain's reward center. This brain region informs you that your brain likes this food and wants you to consume it more often. In the presence of marijuana, significantly more dopamine is released in response to the same amount of sugar-enriched food. So what does all of this mean? Our brain's endogenous marijuana system ordinarily modulates how good a particular food tastes to us; smoking marijuana simply enhances this natural mechanism in the brain.

Our brain's main purpose is to help us survive and pass on our genes. Eating is a critical and necessary behavior that the brain organizes and controls that allows daily survival. Therefore, the brain rewards itself for successfully consuming enough calories to survive by releasing these two powerful neurotransmitters—endorphins and endocannabinoids. As a consequence of the manner in which evolution has shaped the response of our brain to food, overeating of calorie-dense foods has become a major health problem in the developed world. Our brains were shaped by evolution to be very efficient at instructing us to eat, but quite inefficient at stopping us from eating.

Why Does Fat Taste So Good?

One of the best things about the taste of chocolate is its wonderful creamy smoothness. That feeling is due to the presence of fats. In spite of this universal feeling that fatty foods produce on the tongue, scientists have always claimed that we do not actually possess the ability to taste fat. The textbooks only mention our ability to taste sour, salty, sweet, bitter and, rather recently, umami (which is the taste produced by the additive MSG). A recent study demonstrated that humans, and other animals, exhibit a protein on their tongue that can sense the presence of fat. If there is a protein for tasting fat, then there must be a gene responsible for this protein. Indeed, this gene has been identified and it appears as though variations in this gene explain why some people are far more sensitive to fat in their food than others.

The amount of this fat-tasting protein on the tongue varies. If you've inherited a tendency to have fewer of these receptors, then your response to fat is muted and you are more likely to be obese. Obese people do prefer food with higher fat content and consume fat as a larger percentage of their overall calorie intake. Even if you have not inherited this tendency, if you consume lots of fatty foods you will modify the activity of this gene and subsequently make less of the fat-tasting protein. Unfortunately, as a consequence you become less sensitive to the taste of fat and begin to prefer foods that contain higher levels of fat in order to obtain the same pleasurable sensation when eating. Essentially, you start eating more fatty foods but enjoy their taste much less.

WHY IS OBESITY SO HARD TO DEFEAT?

We are all aware that diets high in fat and sugar will lead to obesity. The problem is, fat and sugar are craved like heroin or methamphetamine. Why is this so? The answer is that these foods actually change how the brain functions. Day after day, year after year, the constant bathing of the brain in fats and sugar slowly changes how the DNA in the cells of our brain's feeding center behaves. With these gradual modifications in gene function, our brain circuitry also changes; ultimately, it rewires itself. Eventually we eat more fat and sugar every day in order to feed this ever-more-powerful new reprograming that is evolving inside our brain.

Scientists once assumed that obese people were simply addicted to food in the same manner that someone becomes addicted to heroin—that is, food produces happy, pleasant feelings, and therefore eating lots of food would produce extremely pleasant feelings. Not so. A few years ago scientists discovered just the opposite was true: The brain's reward center decreased its response to eating tasty foods. In obese humans dopamine function becomes significantly impaired in response to many years of poor diet. As a consequence, people consume ever greater quantities of fat and sugar in order to mitigate the diminished rewards that were once experienced by consuming only one scoop of ice cream or a small donut.

Blame It on Your Genes

Are we born destined to become obese? Apparently, yes. Many studies have shown that children who have two obese or overweight parents are four times more likely to become obese themselves. To be considered low risk, the parents of the adolescents needed to be lean, with a body mass index less than 25. When the children in the high-risk group were shown pictures of tasty-looking, high-calorie foods, the dopamine-dependent pleasure centers in their brains became highly activated, especially as compared to the response of the same brain regions in the low-risk children. Children who are destined to become obese apparently inherit a dopamine system that becomes much more excited at the sight of a chocolate milkshake than does the dopamine system in the brain of a child who is not destined to become obese as an adult.

Bugs to the Rescue

Stand naked in front of a mirror. Look closely—really closely! Put on a pair of magic glasses that allows you to see the immense multitude of creatures looking back at you. For every 1 of your big human cells, roughly 100 to 1,000 little bugs live alongside and inside of you. If you were to count all of the cells on and inside of you that are not actually YOU, they would number in the tens of trillions, with approximately

1 million of these microbes living within every square centimeter of your skin! You are never really alone. These little bugs that have hitched their fortunes to you contribute to your good health as well as to your sickness. As our species and theirs evolved, we established some rules to govern our cohabitation, and most of the time everything works out well. But like an unpredictable roommate, these bugs can turn against us and their impact on brain function can be profound because they share our body's exposure to the drugs and foods we consume. Obesity induces an imbalance in the body's intricately choreographed dance with these little creatures. Why? Because during the process of depositing and filling fat cells another cell type, called a macrophage, becomes embedded among our fat cells. Macrophages are part of our body's immune defense system. When they are surrounded by fat cells, these macrophages start releasing chemicals that impair the body's ability to regulate glucose and fat metabolism while also making our bodies insensitive to insulin—this is known as the dreaded metabolic syndrome.

How can we turn off these nasty macrophages? The hero of our story is a cell called an eosinophil. The more of these eosinophils you have in your body, the better able you are to reverse the negative effects of macrophages. One of the most effective signals for inducing your body to produce more eosinophils (and you're not going to like this!) is infection by parasitic worms. After a group of scientists at the University of California at San Francisco infected obese mice on a fatty diet with a parasitic worm, the body fat disappeared and glucose tolerance was restored! I realize that this idea sounds disgusting, but just keep in mind that your new parasitic companion would have lots and lots of company, you would lose lots of weight, and after a little while you would become accustomed to those subtle undulations within your abdomen as the worm grew ever larger while consuming all of your body fat. Fortunately, these scientists also determined that the worm need only spend a week within your gut in order for you to benefit from its ability to activate your eosinophils. Fat farms and health spas would be able to offer some interesting package deals!

This study has some broad implications related to our overly hygienic lifestyle in developed countries that often have the greatest percentage of obese citizens. We co-evolved with many different parasitic species; we still carry many of them around with us all of the time. Thus, inviting into our bodies just one more parasitic worm could become an integral part of a new Paleolithic diet plan.

Okay, if there are trillions of other very small creatures in your body, what are they busy doing right now? Your bacteria, viruses, and fungi are always busy doing quite simple tasks, at least from our perspective—not so much from theirs'. First, they're trying to stay alive as they battle each other for dominance. Second, they're trying to win this continuing battle by replicating themselves as much as possible. In order to do so they require the food that is regularly provided by each meal we consume. Whoever eats more also produces more offspring and wins the battle of survival; this war is waged continuously every day. A shift in the mixture of these bugs can lead to poor health, including heart disease, inflammatory bowel diseases, high cholesterol, obesity, and cancer. The balance of gut bacteria is also thought to influence behavior and the presence of certain mental disorders, such as depression.

Ordinarily we live in harmony with the trillions of little creatures that share our bodies. Thank goodness, since there are so many more of them than us. In general, we'd like them to stay out of our brains, but unfortunately, they rarely follow orders, particularly a one-celled parasite known as *Toxoplasma gondii*. You've heard about this one before because it's been blamed for various illnesses and cancers associated with handling cat litter. *Toxoplasma gondii* is everywhere. Statistically speaking, you and I are both infected but are simply not aware of it. Without a doubt, the presence of *T. gondii* in your brain affects your behavior. Indeed, the evolution of our genus probably owes much to the influence of this parasite in our brains during the past few hundred thousand years. *T. gondii* possesses genes that are capable of causing our brain to greatly increase its production of the neurotransmitter dopamine. People infected with *T. gondii* exhibit many of the symptoms expected of someone whose brain contains far too much dopamine. For example, men infected with *T. gondii* tend to be more extroverted, more aggressive, more suspicious, and more prone to jealousy. In contrast, infected women tend to be more warmhearted and easygoing and much less prone to jealousy or suspicions. However, infected women both attempt and complete suicide more often than women who do not harbor the parasite in their brain.

It is thought that this parasite has been living in the brain, and thus influencing behavior, for as long as the *Homo* genus has existed. Its presence can predispose someone to schizophrenia or drive large groups of infected people to go to war. Did possessing this parasite make it more likely for one group of garrulous people to triumph over another uninfected population? Its continued presence might explain why war is still with us today.

Dieting Versus Exercise: Which Is Best?

The trainer for the NBC show "The Biggest Loser" used to think that more exercise was all that was necessary in order to lose weight. After many years of helping severely obese people lose weight, however, Bob Harper has concluded that exercise is not the key; diet matters most.

Not only is Harper helping his clients to feel better and achieve their personal goals, he is also helping them to live longer, healthier lives. Excess body fat accelerates aging and increases our risk of dying because, as I've already discussed, fat cells produce inflammation. Researchers recently investigated whether diet or exercise most effectively reduced the levels of inflammation in overweight or obese women. After 12 months the scientists concluded that the greatest weight loss and most significant reduction in the level of inflammatory protein reduction came only from dieting. The women who participated in an exercise-only program showed no reduction in inflammatory proteins. Essentially, unless you're a marathon runner or swimmer, the activity of our musculature is not a big player in calorie consumption.

In a recent study, a large group of monkeys, ranging in age from middle-aged to quite elderly, were fed only 70% of their free-feeding diet for about 15 years. Basically, for someone eating a 2,000-calorie per-day diet, this would be about 600 fewer calories per day. As a result of eating just 30% fewer calories, the brains of the monkeys on the restricted diet aged significantly more slowly, developed far fewer age-related diseases, had virtually no indication of diabetes and almost no age-related muscle atrophy, and lived much longer. Most importantly, and consistent with Bob Harper's conclusion, these monkeys did not exercise the weight off; they simply consumed fewer calories.

Simply stated, caloric restriction is the only valid, scientifically proven dietary intervention that can slow the aging process, reduce the risk of cancer, and improve health. It's also much cheaper—you'll save money by eating much less food and paying for fewer tennis shoes, workout clothing, and gym memberships. The sooner one loses the fat, the sooner the brain and body can begin to recover. This risk factor is preventable!

THE JANUS EFFECT OF FOOD

The food we eat must be metabolized, a process that requires the oxygen in the air we breathe. Unfortunately, our most basic acts of survival, breathing and eating, are what age our bodies and our brains. If this sounds like the proverbial damned-if-you-do, damned-if-you-don't scenario, well, it sort of is, and yet somehow our species has managed to survive this challenge for several hundred millennia.

Like most other animals on this planet, we humans acquire energy for our biochemical machinery by breaking down the carbon bonds found in fats, sugars, and proteins and then gobbling as much energy from the process as possible. The fact that we do this so inefficiently means that much of the energy in our food is lost as heat. This process also leaves our cells with leftover carbon atoms. The problem is what to do with all of this carbon waste. More than 2 billion years ago, the solution for a small, independently living single-celled organism, which might have closely resembled our own mitochondria (the furnace that handles almost all of our cells' energy production needs), was to combine these leftover carbons with a readily available gas, oxygen, and to expel the product as a gas called carbon dioxide. Thus, thanks to our current symbiotic relationship with the descendants of these ancient bacteria, our mitochondria, the way our bodies obtain energy to live is as follows: Carbon bonds come into the front end of our feeding tubes in the form of fats, carbohydrates, and proteins; we then extract energy and excrete the residue as carbon dioxide and water vapor.

Because oxygen is also exceedingly toxic to cells, it must be used very carefully and conservatively. Indeed, scientists have recently discovered that the genes that control energy metabolism have been highly conserved across millions of years of evolution, from yeast to humans, and that these genes influence the rate of the aging process. Essentially, the better we negotiate our energy–oxygen exchange with our indwelling mitochondria, the longer and healthier we live as a single individual and as a species. Disrupt the balance in this exchange, and the impact can be harmful.

In general, the hemoglobin in our blood does a decent job of regulating the oxygen levels near the individual cells of our bodies so that those cells have the oxygen they need for respiration, but not too much to kill them outright. These cells have also evolved numerous antioxidant systems that would allow us live to be 115 years old, if we were lucky and ate very, very little food. But most of us are not that lucky, and most of us eat all of the time and just keep on breathing, making ourselves vulnerable to the consequences of oxygen. Thus, our bodies and our brains age more rapidly.

With normal aging, because we insist on eating and breathing, tissue-damaging molecules called *oxygen-free radicals* are formed by our mitochondria. Free radicals are not always harmful, but they become more prevalent with age and may slowly overwhelm our natural antioxidant systems, destroying our neurons and just about every other cell in our bodies. According to another recent discovery, the overproduction of these oxygen-free radicals may encourage cancer cells to metastasize and move around the body. Think about the unbelievable irony of this process: The mitochondrial power plant that resides in quite large numbers in every cell of our bodies is actively injuring those cells by the very process of trying to keep them alive. It turns out that each species' maximum life span may be determined by how many free radicals are produced by the hundreds of mitochondria that live in each of their cells. We are, indeed, our own worst enemy.

PROTECTING THE BRAIN FROM AGING WITH FRUITS AND VEGETABLES

Sometimes scientists tell us things that we're fairly certain we already believe. Still, it's always nice to know that what we believe to be true is in fact true. A group of scientists investigated whether eating fruits and vegetables for 13 years would actually protect against a decline in cognitive abilities that humans commonly experience with normal aging. It does, and this is how they proved it.

The study involved about 2,500 subjects who finished the study and adequately completed all the dietary and cognitive evaluations. The subjects were between the ages of 45 and 60 years old at the beginning of the 13-year study, and each was required to maintain careful and detailed records of their daily diets. The subjects were evaluated at the beginning and end of the study for a variety of cognitive abilities, including verbal memory and higher executive functions such as decision-making and mental flexibility, among many other tests. There is good news and bad news in the results.

First, their diet was composed of a variety of fruits and vegetables, but specifically excluded potatoes, legumes, and dried fruits (each of these foods introduces specific complications that might interfere with the outcome). The adults were divided into groups according to the following diets: folate-rich diets containing both fruits and vegetables, beta-carotene-rich diets containing both fruits and vegetables, vitamin C–rich diets of both fruits and vegetables, and vitamin E–rich diets containing both fruits and vegetables. The individual consumption of specific nutrients—folate, beta-carotene, and vitamins C and E—was also monitored. The subjects were allowed to choose how much of each diet they wished to consume each day; therefore, daily intakes of each nutrient varied. This was allowed in order to more closely reproduce how most of us actually select our daily intakes. At the end of the study, this is what they found. Eating fruits and vegetables has differential and significant beneficial effects on different aspects of brain function. When the specific diets were examined more closely, diets that consisted of only fruits or diets with fruits and vegetables rich in vitamins C and E selectively benefited only verbal memory scores. This test involved being told to remember 48 different words and then recalling them after a delay with distractions. The surprising finding was that eating fruits and vegetables had no significant benefit on other types of tasks that required alternative types of memory, such as learning motor tasks or recognizing familiar objects. Clearly, each component of our diets may influence how well our brain works in unique ways.

Natural antioxidants found in fruits and vegetables, like polyphenols, provide protective effects for the brain through a variety of biological actions. Polyphenols are everywhere in nature; more than 50 different plant species and over 8,000 such compounds have been identified in plant extracts. Obviously, investigating the multiple health benefits of these natural chemicals poses an enormous challenge. Probably the most thoroughly investigated polyphenols are quercetin found in apples, tea, and onions, and resveratrol found in the skin of grapes. Grapes use resveratrol to defend against fungus. Tea contains a number of beneficial chemicals. In neurodegenerative diseases, administration of tea extracts reduced the production of mutant proteins and may prevent neuron cell death in Alzheimer's disease. Although tea is not a cure for Alzheimer's disease, its use is certainly justified given its safety and potential for long-term benefits.

Recently, a friend who has been trying to lose weight for many years indicated that her new diet requires that she eat only meat. When I asked whether she was also eating fruits, she answered that fruits are full of sugar, thus not part of her new healthy diet. This is a common recommendation for many of the new, popular diets—avoid carbohydrates in any form. There are some good arguments to be made about avoiding sugar, but if this approach takes fruits out of your diet, you may be missing important nutrients that might make you healthier in the long term. I want to introduce you to one of these nutrients: ursolic acid.

Ursolic acid is found in apples (mostly in the skin), cranberries, and prunes, as well as in elderflower, basil, bilberries, peppermint, rosemary, thyme, and oregano. Although a considerable number of studies have already documented the ability of this chemical to inhibit the growth of various types of cancer cells, that's not why I want to mention it here. Eating fruits and spices that contain ursolic acid might also enhance brain function and reverse some of the negative effects of obesity on the brain as you get older. Studies have shown that ursolic acid can improve cognitive functioning by increasing your brain and body's sensitivity to insulin. The biological mechanisms have now been fairly well investigated and it appears that ursolic acid is able to correct the errors in metabolism induced by long-term obesity. The real challenge is to discover how many apples, prunes, and cranberries one needs to eat in order to achieve these benefits. Studies on humans have never been performed.

Will you lose weight by eating these fruits? Maybe, it depends on what else you're eating. Will you lose weight avoiding fruits and berries while only eating meat? Yes. However, over the long term, it is unwise to do so. The benefits of an all-meat diet are more immediate than the benefits of eating apples, cranberries, and prunes, because their effects on your health take longer to notice. Essentially, these fad diets have not been around long enough for medical science to determine the long-term risks. Caloric restriction is the only valid, scientifically proven dietary intervention that has been shown to slow the aging process and improve health. The reason we hear so little about this approach is because no one stands to make a profit on all of us eating less food and more apples, cranberries, and prunes.

DON'T FORGET THE SPICE

My grocery store stopped selling an excellent margarita mix because its label states that it contains the preservative sodium benzoate. Sodium benzoate prevents food from molding and can be found in lots of foods and many popular soft drinks. The label on this drink mix claimed that it contained only "natural ingredients." There were complaints from some consumers that inclusion of this preservative violated that claim. Is sodium benzoate truly unnatural? Certainly not! Is it harmful? The answer for sodium benzoate, as for so many ingredients in the foods we consume is always the same: yes and no…and it depends. In order to answer this question, we need to consider the natural source of sodium benzoate: cinnamon. Cinnamon is a spice obtained from the bark of the *Cinnamomum verum* tree. Since antiquity it has had many uses. Moses included it as an ingredient of the holy anointing oil. The Chinese knew it as Gui Zhi and recommended it for its antibacterial and antipyretic properties. Medieval physicians included cinnamon in their preparations to treat arthritis and infections. The widespread use of willow tree bark (and the aspirin-like chemical that was derived from it) for these ailments was still a thousand years into the future.

Cinnamon is metabolized into sodium benzoate. Eating cinnamon significantly elevates the level of sodium benzoate in your brain. A recent study found that eating cinnamon may prevent a variety of age-related neurological disorders. How does this happen? The sodium benzoate produced in the body after eating cinnamon induces significant increases in the levels of a variety of chemicals in the brain called *neurotrophic factors*. These factors stimulate the birth of new neurons in the brain and encourage the survival of existing neurons. These two processes are critical for the maintenance of a healthy brain. During the past decade, many scientific studies have discovered that these neurotrophic factors can prevent, or greatly slow, the progression of a variety of degenerative diseases of the brain, including Alzheimer's and Parkinson's disease. Cinnamon has also been shown to reduce blood sugar levels in people with type II diabetes and reduce cholesterol levels by up to 25%. Thus, cinnamon is good for your brain and body.

Curcumin, derived from the spice turmeric, the powdered rhizome of the medicinal plant *Curcuma longa,* has been used for many centuries throughout Asia and India as a food additive and a traditional herbal remedy. I have published studies showing that curcumin has potent antioxidative and anti-inflammatory proclivities that may be beneficial for patients with either Alzheimer's or Parkinson's disease. Treatments with natural antioxidants and anti-inflammatories through diet or dietary supplements are becoming attractive alternatives. Epidemiological and other research findings strongly indicate that the solution to aging well is exactly what you've heard from your mom: Eat healthy and in moderation; exercise a little and in moderation.

FLAVINOIDS TO THE RESCUE

"Let food be thy medicine and medicine be thy food," said Hippocrates. During the past 2,500 years since the time of Hippocrates, science has made significant progress in understanding how food exerts its beneficial effects on health. We now have solid proof that the foods and beverages that are consumed by humans, in particular those derived from tea leaves, coffee and cocoa beans, celery, grapes, mangos, berries, hops, and other grains, have clearly defined beneficial actions on brain function. While these foods and drinks have quite different chemical compositions, they all contain compounds called flavonoids. Flavonoids are not nutritious, but they are believed to be responsible for the beneficial effects of many foods on the brain.

For many decades the biochemical benefits of flavonoids were attributed to their ability to confer protection from oxygen—they are antioxidants. While flavonoids are capable of acting in this fashion in laboratory experiments, it is unlikely that they can provide this benefit within the brain. The reason is that the flavonoids obtained from the diet do not achieve an adequate level in the brain that would allow them to act as effective antioxidants. So how do they benefit us?

In order to answer this question, scientists have investigated what flavonoids can do when their concentration in the brain is extremely low, at levels that might be achieved by a diet rich in these fruits. The flavonoids directly induce neurons in the brain to become more plastic—that is, more capable of forming new memories. The flavonoids achieve this by directly interacting with specific proteins and enzymes that are critical for learning and memory. They also induce the birth of new neurons, a process that is critical for recovering from injury, exposure to toxins, and the consequences of advanced age, such as increased levels of brain inflammation. Finally, some recent studies have shown that flavonoids actually enhance blood flow to active brain regions.

So how much is enough? Let's consider two of my favorites: wine and chocolate. If you consumed about 200 milliliters (6.7 ounces) of Cabernet Sauvignon or about 50 grams (1.7 ounces) of dark chocolate (71% cocoa powder), you would intake nearly identical quantities of flavonoids, which, fortunately, is now the daily wine intake recommended to produce the most health benefits in a typical adult. When young adult females were given flavonoid-rich chocolate drinks, blood flow to their brain was significantly increased within just 2 hours, and their performance on a complex mental task was greatly improved.

No one is certain whether all flavonoids are capable of producing these benefits. But recent investigations have suggested that it does not matter which type of food provides the flavonoids, only that they are eaten as often as possible. In addition to those edibles mentioned above, studies to date have also identified benefits from black currants, pears, blueberries, strawberries, and grapefruit. One final caveat: No studies have yet proven a true cause-and-effect connection between the lifelong consumption of flavonoid-rich diets and a reversal of age-related deterioration in learning or general mental function. Still, I think that we should all be willing to make a leap of faith that the connection is real and modify our diets accordingly. Such as eating more chocolate!

MORE ON CHOCOLATE AND ITS ACTION IN THE BRAIN

In 1648, according to the diary of English Jesuit Thomas Gage, the women of Chiapas Real arranged for the murder of a certain bishop who forbade them to drink chocolate during mass. In an ironic twist, the pontiff was ultimately found murdered after someone had added poison to his daily cup of chocolate.

Was this an act of blind rage by the women of Chiapas Real or justifiable homicide? For a small percentage of the population, eating chocolate can produce rage, paranoia, and anger that occur without warning. Fortunately, for most of us, this is not the typical reaction to eating chocolate.

In order to understand why chocolate is so enjoyable for some while it induces uncontrollable rage in others, we need to consider the contents of most dark chocolates. Chocolate contains an array of compounds that contribute to the pleasurable sensation of eating it. Many of these compounds are quite psychoactive if they are able to get into our brains. Are they the reason we love chocolate so much? Are they the reason some people fly into fits of anger? The answer to both questions is, of course, yes. However, as is true for so many of the things we eat that affect our brain, it's not all that simple.

Chocolate usually contains fats that may induce the release of endogenous molecules that act similarly to heroin and produce a feeling of euphoria. German researchers reported that drugs that are able to block the actions of this opiate-like chemical produced by eating chocolate prevented the pleasure associated with eating chocolate. Chocolate also contains a small amount of the marijuana-like neurotransmitter called anandamide. Although this molecule can easily cross the blood–brain barrier, the levels in chocolate are probably too low to produce an effect on our mood by itself.

Chocolate contains some estrogen-like compounds, a fact that may explain a recent series of reports showing that men who eat chocolate live longer than men who do not eat chocolate (the effect was not seen for women who have an ample supply of their own estrogen until menopause). However, estrogen is not likely to cause rage, only the urge to shop.

Let's focus on those women of Chiapas Real again. In contrast to its effects on men, women more often claim that chocolate can lift their spirits. In a study of college students and their parents, 14% of sons and fathers and 33% of daughters and mothers met the standard of being substantially addicted to chocolate. Women seem to have very strong cravings for chocolate just prior to and during their menstrual cycle.

Women eat more and crave more foods in the days before the start of their period when progesterone levels are low. This is when premenstrual symptoms tend to appear as well. Chocolate may provide an antidepressant effect during this period. In one study researchers found that women in their 50s often develop a sudden strong craving for chocolate. It turns out that most of the women had just entered menopause and were on a standard form of estrogen replacement therapy consisting of 20 days of estrogen and 10 days of progesterone. The chocolate cravings developed during the days on progesterone. Why?

Chocolate contains magnesium salts, the absence of which in elderly females may be responsible for the common post-menopausal condition known as chocoholism. About 100 milligrams of magnesium salt is sufficient to take away any trace of chocoholism in these women; but who would want to do that? And finally, a standard bar of chocolate contains as many anti-oxidants as a glass of red wine. Clearly, there are many good reasons for men and women to eat chocolate to obtain its indescribably soothing, mellow, and yet euphoric effect.

Okay, what about the anger? How might that happen? Chocolate contains phenethylamine (PEA), a molecule that resembles amphetamine and some of the other psychoactive stimulants. When chocolate is eaten, PEA is rapidly metabolized by the enzyme monoamine oxidase (MAO). Fifty percent of the PEA you consume in a chocolate bar is metabolized within only 10 minutes. Thus very little PEA usually reaches the brain, thus contributing little or no appreciable psychoactive effect without the use of a drug that can inhibit MAO. Could this happen?

Possibly yes. MAO levels are at their lowest level in premenstrual women, which is the time when women most crave the soothing effects of chocolate. In addition, chocolate also contains small amounts of the amino acid tyramine. Tyramine can powerfully induce the release of adrenaline, increase blood pressure and heart rate, and produce nausea and headaches. Usually, the nasty effects of tyramine are prevented because it, too, is metabolized by MAO. You can see the problem: The tyramine and PEA in chocolate may slow each other's metabolism. The consequence is that if both of these chemicals hang around too long in the body, high blood pressure, a fast-beating heart, heightened arousal, racing thoughts, anger, anxiety, and rage would ensue. One rather controversial study claimed that inhibitors of MAO were able to increase PEA levels in the brain by 1,000-fold! That's a lot, and the consequences of this actually happening could be lethal. But the potential exists for some vulnerable people to experience significant shifts in mood after eating chocolate with high cocoa powder levels.

The main point to take away from this discussion about chocolate is that plants, such as the pods from the cocoa tree, contain a complex variety of chemicals that, when considered individually, are not likely to impact our brain function. However, when considered in aggregate, they may exert compound effects throughout the body; some of those effects may be desirable, while others may not. Chocolate is an excellent example of how difficult it is to differentiate food from drugs.

CHAPTER 3

MEMORIES, MAGIC, AND A MAJOR ADDICTION

W hat causes memory loss in patients with Alzheimer's disease? Why did witches once believe that they could fly? Why is it so hard to stop smoking? The answers to these questions can be found by understanding the function of acetylcholine, a neurotransmitter chemical that exists almost everywhere in nature.

Acetylcholine was discovered by the pharmacologist Otto Loewi a couple days after Easter Sunday in 1920 while working at University College, London. His equipment was simple but his insights demonstrated true genius. Loewi shared the Nobel Prize for Physiology or Medicine in 1936 with Henry Dale, also a pharmacologist, for their work on chemical neurotransmission. Acetylcholine has been found in both uni- and multicellular organisms, including the bacterium *Pseudomonas fluorescens*, isolated from the juice of fermenting cucumbers, as well as in the blue-green algae, *Oscillatoria agardhii*, where it may be involved with photosynthesis. Acetylcholine stimulates silk production in spiders and limb regeneration in salamanders. In humans, acetylcholine enables movement by stimulating the muscles to contract, and it plays an important role in the action of the parasympathetic and sympathetic nervous systems, which are part of the autonomic nervous system (ANS). The ANS maintains homeostasis, or a balance of forces or equilibrium, for your entire body. Among other functions, it controls the rate at which your heart beats, how fast you breathe, how much saliva your mouth is making, the rate of movement of material in your gut, your ability to initiate urination, how much you are perspiring, the size of your pupils, and the degree of visible sexual excitation you might experience. Within the human brain are numerous acetylcholine pathways that influence the function of the cortex, hippocampus, and many other regions. Within these various regions, the actions of acetylcholine enable you to learn and remember, to regulate your attention and mood, and to control how well you can move. Thus, anything that affects the function of acetylcholine neurons has the potential to affect all of these brain and body functions. That "anything" could be a certain drug or a disease.

A CASE IN POINT: ALZHEIMER'S DISEASE

Sometimes we can learn much about the role of a particular neurotransmitter system by investigating what happens when it is injured or diseased. In the brains of people with Alzheimer's disease, for example, acetylcholine neurons that project into the hippocampus and cortex very slowly die. The effects of this neuronal death have been the subject of research in my laboratory for more than 25 years. The loss of normal acetylcholine function in the cortex may be why patients with Alzheimer's disease have difficulty paying attention to their environment. The loss of acetylcholine projections to the amygdala, part of the brain's limbic system, may underlie the emotional instability, such as irritability and paranoia, that is sometimes observed in these patients. And the loss of acetylcholine projections into the hippocampus may underlie the profoundly debilitating memory loss that is the major hallmark of this disease.

Let me illustrate the effect of at least one of these losses by first describing the role of acetylcholine in the cortex of a normal brain (yours). Imagine that, using an electroencephalogram (EEG), I have attached some electrodes to the front half of your head to record the electrical activity occurring inside your brain. Next, I calmly inform you that as soon as I ring a bell (at the point in time shown by the number 1 in Figure 3.1), a masked gunman will enter the room and start shooting. You must also believe that I'm telling the truth for this to work. Okay, now I ring the bell. Take a

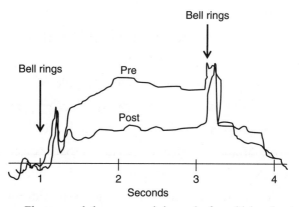

Figure 3.1. Electroencephalogram recorded over the frontal lobes showing the presence of an "anticipation wave" with an intact acetylcholine system (labeled "Pre") and without a functioning acetylcholine system (labeled "Post"). The sharp vertical spikes are associated with a bell ringing at the beginning and end of the recording.

look at the EEG recording labeled "Pre" in the figure. It shows that an electrical wave quickly appears within the frontal lobes of your brain that began as soon as I rang the bell. The bell ringing causes those sharp spikes prior to the formation of the wave. This electrical pattern, also known as an EEG wave, will continue to live in your brain until one of two things happens: Either someone runs into the room with a gun (at the point in time shown by the number 3) or the bell rings again and you decide nothing is going to happen after all. At that point, the EEG wave will disappear. This "pre-wave" indicates that you were paying close attention to what you thought was about to happen. It is an expression of your brain experiencing anticipation.

Experiments in my laboratory and in others have demonstrated that the appearance of this wave of electrical activity

requires the normal function of acetylcholine within your frontal cortex. If the acetylcholine neurons that project into your
frontal cortex are destroyed, then this wave cannot fully form
and you will have great difficulty paying attention to important
things, such as the impending appearance of a masked gunman.
An example of such a wave is labeled "Post" in the figure. In
this case, the absence of acetylcholine does not allow the wave
to fully develop. This research has demonstrated that acetylcholine's job is to instruct the neurons in your frontal cortex to pay
attention to important information and be vigilant to impending danger. If acetylcholine function is impaired, this ability is
lost. These results provide valuable insight into why patients
with Alzheimer's disease have trouble paying attention to things
that might be important, or even harmful, to them. Indeed, during the later stages of their disease, when most of these acetylcholine neurons have disappeared, patients have difficulty paying
attention to anything at all.

Keep the Aluminum Cookware—It Does Not Cause Alzheimer's Disease

Aluminum is everywhere around us all of the time. It is the
most abundant metal in the Earth's crust. Yet, somehow, we
have become fearful of it when it is used as cookware or as cans
for beer or sodas. No life form uses aluminum for any biological process. The reason is that aluminum is highly reactive and
easily combines with other metals and oxygen to form hundreds
of different minerals. Aluminum, in scientific terms, is not

bioavailable to humans—usually. It all depends on what chemical form the aluminum takes on. Usually, because aluminum is so tightly bound within minerals, animals have no chance to absorb it into their tissues.

Plants do not use aluminum, but they are capable of absorbing it. Grains harvested to make bread and cereals often contain a few parts per million of aluminum. This aluminum exists within a bioavailable form that we humans can absorb into our bodies. Animals that eat plants have concentrations of aluminum in their tissues, too. Thus, meats obtained from cows may contain up to 1,000 parts per million of aluminum. This is where things get a little dicey. Are we at risk from the aluminum in our diet? It depends entirely on how much you consume. Some people are vulnerable to its presence in the body. Aluminum has also been found in the brains of patients who have died with Alzheimer's disease. Although this seems suspicious, aluminum salts will deposit in any soft tissue that has cell loss due to injury or degeneration. Thus, aluminum salts also deposit in the hearts of people with coronary disease. Aluminum does not cause Alzheimer's disease.

What about deodorants? The aluminum salts used in these products do one thing—they irritate our sweat glands to the point that they swell and close the pores that allow perspiration to reach the surface of our skin. The real risk from deodorants comes from using sprays that produce a cloud of aluminum salts that can be inadvertently inhaled. Thus, keep using your aluminum cookware—they pose no risk to health. The real risk comes from the food we cook in those pots and pans.

ACETYLCHOLINE PRODUCTION
AND RELEASE

Sometimes, the severity of the cognitive symptoms in Alzheimer's disease can be reduced, at least to some degree, by drugs and dietary nutrients that enhance the function of acetylcholine neurons in the brain. To understand how this is possible, we need to look at how acetylcholine is produced in the brain in the first place.

Neurons synthesize acetylcholine from choline, which is obtained from the diet, and from acetyl groups that originate in mitochondria from the metabolism of sugar. Here is yet another example of the importance of sugar for your brain's normal function. The synthesis of acetylcholine occurs within the cytoplasm of your neurons, and the product is stored in synaptic vesicles, those small, round packets that neurons release to communicate with each other. Neurons pay a lot of attention to the shelf life of their neurotransmitters; they prefer to release the most recently produced neurotransmitter molecules first. As you can see, neurons do not behave like your local grocer; they do not rotate their stock. This means that the freshest products (the most recently produced acetylcholine molecules) are released first, thus guaranteeing that the communication between neurons is successful.

Many health food stores in malls across America sell choline powder to gullible customers, claiming that consuming more choline will somehow enable their brains to make more acetylcholine. Given the vital role of acetylcholine in learning and memory, this is an appealing claim. Regrettably, it has no basis in fact. For adults, the brain responds only to deficits, not surpluses, in the diet. It has a ready source of choline in the diet or stored in the liver and, in fact, never develops a deficit in choline, even in patients with Alzheimer's disease. Thus, consuming extra choline does not induce your brain to make more acetylcholine. Instead, it only results in a gaseous byproduct that you exhale and that smells like rotting fish. Rather than enhancing your cognitive abilities, choline supplements merely generate a terrible case of bad breath.

Once released, the action of acetylcholine within the synapse is terminated or inactivated by an enzyme called acetylcholinesterase at the rate of approximately 25,000 molecules per second. Thus, even the partial inhibition of this enzyme's activity has a profound effect on synaptic levels of acetylcholine. Many different drugs are capable of inhibiting this enzyme, including some nerve gases that cause synaptic levels of acetylcholine to rise too high and that are therefore highly poisonous, as well as some drugs that cause the level to rise just enough to be clinically beneficial. Physostigmine, for example, is currently being given to patients with Alzheimer's disease to improve their ability to pay attention or remember the day's events, although sadly, its benefits tend to be very limited and they do not alter the ultimate course of the disease. Nonetheless, what the contrasting effects of these drugs have taught neuroscientists is that a little extra acetylcholine in the synaptic cleft between neurons seems to improve our thinking abilities, whereas too much acetylcholine can be lethal.

It's worth considering what would happen if a neuron could not release acetylcholine at all. The botulinum toxin from the *Clostridium botulinum* bacteria that sometimes forms in the foods we eat can inhibit the release of acetylcholine from nerve terminals. Fortunately for your brain, this toxin cannot cross the blood–brain barrier. But unfortunately, there's more to you than just your brain. Botulinum toxin can significantly impair the ability of your vagus nerve to control your breathing. Your vagus nerve is responsible for causing the contraction of your diaphragm muscle to pull air into your lungs (see Figure 3.2). However, if your brain cannot

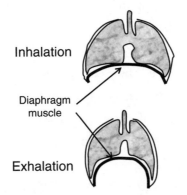

Figure 3.2. The release of acetylcholine onto the diaphragm muscle causes it to contract and pull air into the lungs (inspiration). The relaxation of this muscle allows air to leave the lungs (expiration).

communicate with your diaphragm via the release of acetylcholine from the vagus nerve, then you will stop breathing and die. The botulinum toxin is exceptionally potent; 1 gram is sufficient to kill approximately 350,000 people!

Once released into the synapse, the neurotransmitter acetylcholine can act on two quite different protein receptors that have been designated, as have most receptors, according to the compounds that were originally used to study them—in this case, muscarine and nicotine. Most of the acetylcholine (or "cholinergic") receptors in the brain are the muscarinic subtype, whereas less than 10% are nicotinic. Both types of receptors have been found in peanut worms (whose fossils date back a half-billion years), spoon worms, leeches, and earthworms. There is no evidence that these two receptors are related or share a common evolutionary history: They differ in size, structure, and mechanism of action; yet they both respond to acetylcholine.

Moreover, their response to different drugs tells us something important about the role that these two different acetylcholine receptors play in the brain and the body. Some drugs block, or antagonize, these receptors, whereas other drugs enhance, or stimulate (i.e., act as agonists of), them. Let's now look at several types of drugs to see what their actions reveal about the function of these receptors.

ANTAGONIZING ACETYLCHOLINE

Curare, found in a resinous extract of the plants *Chondrodendron tomentosum* and *Strychnos toxifera*, from the Orinoco and Amazon basins in South America, is an antagonist at nicotinic acetylcholine receptors. Curare does not cross the blood–brain barrier; therefore, its actions are expressed only outside of the brain at the neuromuscular junction where neurons control muscles. Curare is extremely lethal for one simple reason—it blocks the nicotinic receptors located on the diaphragm; therefore, death from curare results from asphyxiation. Imagine you've been shot by a curare-tipped arrow: You'd be awake, fully aware of having been shot, yet completely unable to move, speak, or, ultimately, breathe.

The naturally occurring drugs atropine and scopolamine have a different sort of antagonistic effect: They block the muscarinic subtype of acetylcholine receptors. As a result, they impair our ability to form new memories and produce considerable mental confusion and drowsiness. At high doses, atropine and scopolamine can be lethal.

Several plants contain atropine and scopolamine, including henbane (*Hyoscyamus niger*), jimson weed (*Datura stramonium*), and mandrake (*Mandragora officinarum*). The "bane" part of henbane refers to an archaic Old English word for death; according to legend, local farmers noticed that their hens and roosters did not live long after eating this plant. Another plant, the "deadly nightshade," or *Atropa belladonna*, was given its name by the botanist Carl von Linné in the 18th century to signify its deadly nature. He derived the genus name from one of the Greek fates, Atropos, who cut the thread of life at the appointed time—she was death.

Poets and writers have long been aware of the lethal effects of these plants and have often incorporated them into their stories. For example, consider Shakespeare's tragedy *Hamlet*: King Hamlet of Denmark dies suddenly, ostensibly from snakebite, and a few weeks later, his brother Claudius marries the king's widow, Queen Gertrude. The ghost of the king appears before his son, Prince Hamlet, and reveals that Claudius killed him by pouring into his ear the contents of an ampoule of henbane. In Act I, Scene 5, we find the ghost speaking to Hamlet:

Sleeping within mine orchard, My custom always in the afternoon,
> Upon my secure hour thy uncle stole,
> With juice of cursed hebona [henbane] in a vial,
> And in the porches of mine ears did pour
> The leperous distilment; whose effect
> Holds such as enmity with blood of man.

Enmity indeed!

How did scopolamine and atropine, both components of henbane, kill King Hamlet? To answer this question, let's return to the autonomic nervous system. Recall the functions of the ANS that I mentioned previously. For example, it controls heart and breathing rate, intestinal motility, pupil dilation, salivation, and perspiration. The two major components of the ANS, the parasympathetic and sympathetic nervous systems (see Figure 3.3), essentially function in competition with each

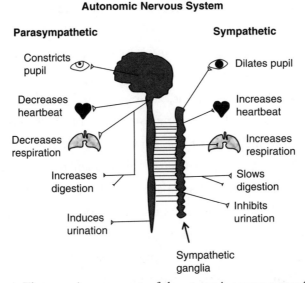

Figure 3.3. The two major components of the autonomic nervous system (ANS). The parasympathetic neurons release acetylcholine; the sympathetic neurons release norepinephrine. These two systems provide a balance of control of the function of the organs and structures shown.

other to maintain a balance so that your heart does not beat too fast or too slowly, you do not breathe too quickly or slowly, the contents of your gut do not move too fast or too slowly, and so forth. When the parasympathetic nervous system is in control, it slows your heart rate, slows your breathing, constricts the pupils of your eyes, increases the production of saliva in your mouth, and so forth. When the sympathetic nervous system is in control, it increases your heart rate, increases your respiration rate, dilates the pupils of your eyes, reduces salivation (leaving you with a dry, metallic taste in your mouth), and so forth. This careful dance between these two competing neural systems is choreographed by your brain, but you are usually not aware of it. However, when something disturbs this balance, such as scopolamine, you become very aware that something is wrong.

Recall that scopolamine, an ingredient in henbane, blocks muscarinic acetylcholine receptors. This blockade essentially removes the influence of the parasympathetic nervous system on the body. In the absence of this influence, the balance of forces is upset and the sympathetic nervous system gains the upper hand. Thus, your heart rate increases, your pupils dilate, salivation stops, your ability to urinate is impaired, and you become constipated; overall, things get very uncomfortable. But none of this is directly lethal (unless the constipation makes one commit suicide). If you do die from an overdose of henbane, it is believed to result from either a complex series of events in your brain that lead to the loss of control of your diaphragm, causing death from asphyxiation, or from cardiac arrest. This is why the deadly nightshade is so deadly and how Shakespeare chose to kill King Hamlet with henbane.

An even earlier literary reference to the toxic effects of extracts from these types of plants appeared in Homer's *Odyssey*. Odysseus, the legendary king of Ithaca and hero of the poem, was advised to defend himself against the sorceress Circe's poison by eating a "moly," which historians think refers to an extract of *Galanthus nivalis,* or snowdrop, a plant similar to henbane. Among the first bulbs to bloom in spring, the snowdrop contains galanthamine, which can inhibit the enzyme acetylcholinesterase, much like physostigmine. By inhibiting acetylcholinesterase, the moly would increase the amount of acetylcholine in the synapse. The additional acetylcholine would be able to compete successfully with the poison for the acetylcholine receptor and prevent death. During Homer's time, a moly might have been a common antidote against poisonous plants containing scopolamine-like drugs. Ironically, extracts from scopolamine-containing plants, like the *Datura*, may also have been used as antidotes to poisoning from eating the snowdrop plant, proving correct once again the words of the Roman poet Lucretius, "One man's poison is another man's antidote."

Simply stated, it is just as dangerous to have too much acetylcholine in the synapse as it is to have too little. During World War II, German chemical companies produced nerve gases that were based on the action of the snowdrop plant and thus were very potent inhibitors of the acetylcholinesterase enzyme. During battle, these gases were designed to be sprayed into the air and then inhaled by soldiers, who would quickly become unable to walk or breathe and would ultimately die. Just as the Greeks seem to have discovered two millennia earlier, the soldiers could defend themselves against this poison by injecting themselves with extracts from the *Datura stramonium* plant. But timing was everything: The soldiers could safely inject the extracts only if they suspected imminent exposure to a nerve gas. Otherwise, the use of this antidote could backfire if no gas attack occurred. Imagine an entire brigade of soldiers infused with scopolamine: They would be fully amnesic, unable to urinate, and mentally confused—not exactly the characteristics of an effective combat unit. Indeed, this is exactly what may have led to the defeat of Marc Antony's army by the Parthians in 36 BCE.

Many of the most effective insecticides available today are based on the same biochemical mechanism of the nerve gases—that is, the potent inhibition of the enzyme acetylcholinesterase. These chemicals are effective as insecticides because insects, who share our evolutionary history on this planet, are also vulnerable to having too much acetylcholine in their synapses.

VOODOO DOLLS, HALLUCINATIONS, AND BEAUTY

This seems as good a place as any to touch on the truly weird to highlight other details relating to antagonists of muscarinic acetylcholine receptors. Voodoo death and the creation of zombies, although not completely well understood as phenomena, are a great illustration of the workings of the ANS. Voodoo itself is a complex religion derived from West African polytheism and is practiced primarily in Haiti. I wish to focus on that famous effigy of vengeance that most people associate with the term: the voodoo doll, into which one person sticks spikes or pins as part of a curse on another person. For people who truly believe in the power of the voodoo doll, the fear that this curse generates in the victim is usually quite powerful. The physiological expressions of this fear result from the extreme activation of the sympathetic nervous system. The unfortunate victim begins to experience uncomfortable heart palpitations, sweating, dry mouth, and heavy breathing that leads to a loss of carbon dioxide, and, as a consequence, lightheadedness. This physical condition plays into the person's fear and expectations of what should be happening as a result of this curse; these thoughts produce more fear and more sympathetic ANS activation.

Unless the person suffers a heart attack resulting from some sort of underlying, undiagnosed heart condition, this extremely fearful experience is not usually lethal. Instead, the excessive activation of the sympathetic nervous system triggers a compensatory reflex called the baroreceptor reflex, which results in an abrupt drop in heart rate called reflex bradycardia (meaning slow heart). Therefore, the cursed victim is not really frightened to death; rather, a deathlike state comes when the sympathetic ANS ultimately turns off, and there is a rebound of equal and opposite magnitude by the parasympathetic ANS. As the parasympathetic system controls more and more of the victim's bodily functions, the heart rate slows way down, and the person will slowly lose consciousness. In this state, the unlucky victim of the voodoo curse might appear to be dead. According to legend, some victims have even been buried while still alive, leading to fairly common myths about the dead rising from their graves, not looking too well, and certainly annoyed by the ugliness that was just perpetrated upon them—obviously, the makings of a great horror movie and everlasting legend.

Fortunately, there is some fascinating pharmacology to take from the voodoo death legends. Most legends talk about a potion containing extracts from jimson weed, *Datura stramonium* (also called the zombie cucumber), which contains scopolamine. How would scopolamine help the victim of a zombie curse? Scopolamine would reduce the influence of the parasympathetic nervous system and prevent the victim from slipping into a zombie-like state.

The actions of scopolamine in the brain are rather complex. For example, low doses produce amnesia and activation of the sympathetic nervous system. They also can produce an array of peripheral side effects that are nicely exemplified by the following story, published in 1980. Police in New York City were finding men wandering around the Central Park area without their pants and their wallets and with no idea of what had happened to them during the previous few hours. The men could see and hear normally and safely avoid objects such as moving cars, dogs, and puzzled tourists. Their mouths were quite dry, and they had dilated pupils and very full bladders that they could not empty. These are all the symptoms of scopolamine ingestion. Ultimately, it was discovered that the men had recently visited prostitutes in the area and had been given a drink containing scopolamine, which had been stolen from a local pharmacy.

Higher doses of scopolamine, on the other hand, can produce visual and auditory hallucinations. The original witches' flying ointment, so called because of its reputed use by medieval witches, was probably an herbal recipe that contained extracts from the *Datura* and *Mandragora* plants, as well as poplar leaves and fireplace soot, all of which were held together with animal fat or clove oil. In a ritual performed in the nude, the witches would rub the ointment on their foreheads, wrists, hands, or feet. According to Abramelin the Mage (1362–1460), a Jew from Wurzburg, Germany, who wrote a series of books on magic and the occult, the women would also "anoint a staff and ride on it...or anoint themselves under the arms and in other hairy places." Their experiences may underlie the origination of stories about witches flying on broomsticks. By anointing "a staff" with the ointment and then riding on it naked, they would inevitably rub the ointment into the mucous membrane of their labia, which would ensure a speedy absorption of the lipid-soluble active ingredients of the plants in the ointment. The sensation produced by sufficient doses of these plant extracts would include both visual hallucinations and a floating, lightheaded feeling; it's not hard to appreciate why these women might have reported an experience similar to flying through the sky while straddling their broomsticks.

These women likely had one thing in common with the Central Park men: They were effectively high on scopolamine. Although no one knows just how scopolamine is able to produce its complex psychoactive effects, those effects are clearly influenced by the dose of scopolamine consumed and by the number and location of muscarinic receptors within the brain that are antagonized. Ophthalmologists use scopolamine for clinical purposes—as an antagonist to block the muscarinic receptors expressed on the smooth muscles that encircle the iris of the eye and to allow the pupils to dilate, thus enabling these doctors to examine the interior of a patient's eyes. There may be another benefit as well, if the patient could see well enough to take advantage of it upon leaving the examination room: Those dilated pupils, unconsciously interpreted to indicate excitement, can be a real turn-on to other people. Indeed, people tend to rate others with dilated pupils as being more attractive and interesting. Von Linné knew this when he gave the species name of "belladonna," or beautiful woman, to one of the plants that produce scopolamine. Even today, products containing extracts of the *Atropa belladonna* plant are sold to women who want to be seen as beautiful and who use these extracts to dilate their eyes. Unfortunately, pupil dilation impairs vision and makes the user quite photophobic; it can also cause profound amnesia. Taken together, however, these multiple conditions might be seen as advantageous by a less attractive suitor.

ENHANCING ACETYLCHOLINE WITH A NUT AND A MUSHROOM

Let's now turn away from the actions of drugs that are antagonists at the muscarinic acetylcholine receptors to consider drugs that are agonists (i.e., stimulants) at this receptor. Arecoline is one such agonist, found in the nut of the areca palm tree (*Areca catechu*) of Asia. The nut is used as a mild euphoriant and antitussive (cough suppressant) throughout Southeast Asia. These effects indicate that arecoline is probably, at the very least, effectively stimulating the muscarinic acetylcholine receptors within the limbic (emotional) system and coughing centers of the brain.

The nut is often eaten wrapped in a leaf from the betel pepper tree (*Piper betle*), together with a piece of limestone; the presence of this bicarbonate-releasing stone increases the pH in the mouth and accelerates the absorption of arecoline and guvacoline from the nut. Some component of the nut is also converted into a bright red pigment that makes saliva become red and stains the teeth. After you've eaten this nut, your body converts some of it into a drug called guvacine, which is a potent enhancer of the neurotransmitter gamma-aminobutyric acid (GABA), the brain's principal inhibitory transmitter molecule. Therefore, the two-fold effect of consuming the Betel nut would be an enhancement of the inhibitory action of GABA throughout the brain similar to that produced by a barbiturate or alcohol, and stimulation of the acetylcholine receptor. For reasons that are not well understood, these combined effects produce feelings of happiness and well-being. These pleasurable feelings are probably the basis for the nut's popularity in Southeast Asia.

Feelings of happiness and well-being can be produced by another drug, muscarine, which also acts by stimulating acetylcholine receptors in the brain and body. Muscarine is present in the mushroom *Amanita muscaria*, which is very brightly colored and appears to be dotted with cottage cheese on its surface (Figure 3.4). Eating this mushroom can also produce hallucinations, although its actual hallucinogenic constituent has not yet been conclusively determined. A typical hallucinogenic dose is about one to three dried mushrooms, depending on their size and growing conditions. The hallucinations are quite interesting. People report that normal objects appear bigger or smaller than they truly are; this is called macropsia or micropsia, respectively. The author Lewis Carroll was clearly aware of the perceptual changes produced by eating this mushroom, having

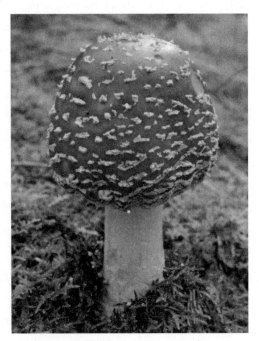

Figure 3.4. The *Amanita muscaria* mushroom.

incorporated them into his book, *Alice in Wonderland*. Carroll may have become familiar with these mushrooms through his close friendship with the famous mycologist (someone who studies fungi), Mordecai Cooke.

The mushrooms also cause sleepiness and then delirium, so at the very least, they probably interfere with the function of acetylcholine neurons within the cortex. Upon waking, people claim to feel very excited and aggressive for 3 to 4 hours and able to perform extraordinary physical feats. These symptoms are consistent with an overactive sympathetic nervous system: Reduced in activity while the contents of the mushroom are in the body, the sympathetic nervous system rebounds in activity after the drug is excreted.

Petroglyphs found in 1968 in North Africa suggest the existence of a 12,000-year-old cult that is thought to have used the *Amanita muscaria* mushroom in religious rituals. The Amanita mushroom was also a popular recreational and ritualistic drug among people living in northern Europe. But perhaps its most memorable use was by the Vikings, whose rather unpleasant behaviors during their invasion of Ireland in the eighth century CE were described as "berserksgang" in the Irish poem "Fury of the Norsemen." From this poem, which includes the phrase "O Lord Deliver Us," you can get a clear idea of what happens when the brain is exposed to the contents of the *Amanita muscaria* mushroom. Its psychoactive ingredients must be quite stable in the body and quite resistant to digestive enzymes because they can be isolated from urine and reused! They will "last" through approximately four consecutive users, as long as those users do not mind drinking someone else's urine. Evidently, the Vikings did not mind.

The mushroom was also known as "fly agaric" because of its ability to attract and kill flies. Flies also have muscarinic acetylcholine receptors on their neurons; after they ingest parts of the mushroom, the overstimulation of these receptors is apparently sufficient to kill them. But even if they somehow survive that fate, they are likely still doomed because of the actions of the mushroom on their retinas, which contain muscarinic acetylcholine receptors as well. After dining on mushroom pieces, the flies may become so visually impaired as to be vulnerable to a carefully aimed boot.

NICOTINE

And what about substances that act as agonists at the nicotinic acetylcholine receptor? At least two may be found in a fruit in your local grocery store. The chemicals punicalin and punicalagin are contained in the rind of the pomegranate, *Punica granatum*; the level of these chemicals is quite high and toxic, although pomegranate seeds are, of course, safe to eat. Another nicotinic agonist, cytosine, is from a more obscure source. It is contained in the seeds of the mescal bean, *Sophora secundiflora*, which was discovered in Central America in archaeological sites dating to 8,000 years ago. The seeds are roasted over a fire and chewed to produce stimulation. The Mescalero Indians also added the beans to beer, whereas the Kickapoo Indians mixed it with tobacco leaves; this mixture was then used to treat earaches.

But by far one of the best-studied agonists of the nicotinic acetylcholine receptor is nicotine. It occurs in more than 64 species of plants around the world, including the well-known tobacco plant, which likely uses nicotine as a defense against insects that express nicotine receptors in their body and are therefore vulnerable to its toxicity.

Tobacco was first used to treat persistent headaches, colds, and abscesses or sores on the head. Tobacco enemas were used to treat flatulence, and even more surprising, the smoke was once inhaled deeply to lessen bad coughs. In 1560, Jean Nicot (then the French ambassador to Portugal) sent some tobacco to Catherine de Medici, who was then queen to Henry II of France; she reported that it helped treat her migraines. The plant initially was given the title of "herbe sainte," or holy plant, and then later was dubbed "Herba Regina," the queen's herb. Nicot got the credit for the discovery and Von Linné named the genus *Nicotiana* in his honor. Despite all this royal glory, in the 1890s the U.S. pharmacopeia dropped nicotine from its list of useful therapeutic agents.

A cigarette made from tobacco will contain about 1 to 2 milligrams of nicotine. Because nicotine is quite volatile and heat labile, only about 20% of it is actually inhaled into the body. However, because of its exceptional lipid solubility, at least 90% of the inhaled nicotine is absorbed into the body. Nicotine can also be rapidly absorbed by the mouth or intact skin. Once the smoke is inhaled, absorption by the lungs and transport to the brain occurs within 2 to 7 seconds. This makes smoking tobacco as efficient as an intravenous injection in getting nicotine to its site of action within the brain. This speed of entry into the body may also explain why nicotine is so toxic. Sixty milligrams is considered a lethal dose for a human; death takes only a few minutes to occur and results from a loss of control of the nicotinic receptors on the diaphragm muscles.

Nicotine affects cortical function in a complex dose-dependent fashion. Low doses tend to activate the left hemisphere and produce mental stimulation and a feeling of arousal, whereas high doses tend to activate the right hemisphere more strongly and are associated with the sedative effects of nicotine. Therefore, when doing boring tasks, you could take a low dose of nicotine by, say, smoking one cigarette and could increase your subjective feelings of arousal and attention. In contrast, during anxious or stressful situations, you could take a high dose of nicotine by chain-smoking and may actually reduce your stress by activating the right hemisphere and producing a bit of sedation. These findings nicely demonstrate the competing roles of nicotine receptors in the two hemispheres and tell us something profound about how the two halves of the brain normally function to produce a balance of emotions, attention, and arousal. Moreover, 60% of adults diagnosed with attention-deficit/hyperactivity disorder smoke cigarettes as compared to less than 30% of the rest of the population, another interesting finding indicating that acetylcholine nicotinic receptors play an important role in paying attention.

Why is smoking so difficult to give up? Smoking produces a powerful rewarding feeling in the brain. Nicotine is the most addictive drug currently used by humans. It produces a dose-related euphoria that is most pronounced following overnight abstinence. Essentially, it provides its greatest pleasure with its first use of each day and re-addicts the user every morning. This may explain why heavy smokers enjoy lighting up as soon as they awaken in the morning. This is a common response of the brain to the absence of various chemicals that we consume; the reintroduction of a drug or nutrient after a prolonged delay produces a bigger effect. For example, food always tastes better when we're hungry. The sensitivity of the sensory neurons in our taste buds on the tongue is increased by hunger. Thus, if you're not a good cook, make your dinner guests wait an extra long time before serving the meal—your cooking will taste better to them. But if you're a dreadful cook, encourage your guests to smoke—this will tend to deaden their tastes buds.

After their initial morning smoke, and throughout the rest of the day, smokers carefully, and probably unconsciously, control the amount of nicotine that reaches their brain by altering the number of cigarettes they use per hour, the rate at which they take a puff, and the volume of their inhalation. This careful regulation may optimize the amount of stimulation to the acetylcholine nicotinic receptor and the balance of right versus left cortical activation to balance the level of stimulation and sedation. People with serious mental illness often are heavy smokers. They may be using nicotine to balance the activity between their two hemispheres and thereby lessen the severity of their symptoms. This potentially positive aspect of smoking may explain why, in 1948, the *Journal of the American Medical Association* stated that "from a psychological point of view, in all probability more can be said in behalf of smoking as a form of escape from tension than against it."

Smoking also influences how your brain experiences food. As if there weren't enough to be concerned about for a smoker, two recent studies have identified some interesting risks and benefits of combining smoking with the consumption of certain foods, including cheese, beer, wine (due to the presence of Resveratrol), turmeric, fava beans, and pickles.

Many decades ago, when tricyclic antidepressant drugs were introduced to the market, they presented some nasty side effects, including death, when the patients consumed any of these foods. The side effect became known as the "cheese effect." The "cheese effect" is due to the ability of these antidepressant drugs to block the enzyme monoamine oxidase (MAO) and the fact that cheese, beer, wine, and the other foods contain high levels of the amino acid tyramine. Ordinarily, tyramine is easily metabolized and inactivated in the body and brain by MAO. Unfortunately, when MAO is inhibited, the consequences of consuming these foods include wild fluctuations in blood pressure, nausea, headache, rash, dizziness, heart palpitations, and vomiting.

Smoking inhibits MAO. The more a person smokes, the greater the inhibition of this critical enzyme throughout the body. You can easily see the potential problems that might arise when a smoker decides to have a glass of wine or beer with their cheese and crackers. Suddenly, you become very nauseous and your heart feels as though it's going to pop out of your chest. Your first thought, of course, is that there's something wrong with the food and you begin to question the culinary skills of your host.

The interesting and rather complex interaction between smoking and eating cheese does not end with these sickly feelings. In contrast to its effects on MAO, smoking actually activates an enzyme in the brain that is responsible for converting tyramine into the neurotransmitter dopamine. The simplest way to explain the purpose of dopamine is to say that it is responsible for your being able to feel pleasure. Indeed, neuroscientists have believed for many years that virtually everything humans enjoy somehow involves triggering the release of dopamine in our brain's pleasure centers. Nicotine has also been found to trigger the release of dopamine.

Taken together, these discoveries suggest that smokers can expect some quite interesting chemical reactions to develop in their bodies at the next wine and cheese party they attend. The consequences of the nicotine and tobacco smoke (both of which seem to play different roles in this process) would act together to produce additional dopamine from the contents of the diet and, additionally, to induce the brain to release that surplus dopamine within the brain's pleasure centers. A double-whammy of pleasure! Smoking and eating cheese at the same time is therefore simultaneously more rewarding, and more dangerous.

Today, our perception of nicotine has been altered prin-cipally by the consequences of using the "vehicle" for nico-tine administration, the tobacco plant. In the United States alone, tobacco use causes almost one death every minute, or the equivalent of four major airline crashes daily, similar to what occurred on September 11, 2001. If we had to witness that tragedy every day, just imagine the public outcry for greater federal control of tobacco. Sadly, because of politics and the fact that tobacco sales (and their taxes) are such a boon to the U.S. economy, this is not likely to ever occur to the degree of banning these sales completely. Meanwhile, people will continue to die from tobacco use and will do so one at a time, at home or in a hospital room, not in large groups on the evening news.

CHAPTER 4

EUPHORIA, DEPRESSION, AND MADNESS

an the function of just one small group of chemicals really determine whether you are happy or sad? The two neurotransmitters that are considered in this chapter, dopamine and norepinephrine, are chemicals called catecholamines that may do exactly that and much more. Catecholamines occur extensively throughout nature and have been identified in insects, crustaceans, arachnids (spiders), and primates. We know a lot about these neurotransmitters in the human brain primarily because so many drugs and nutrients have been discovered that can modify their function. This chapter looks at some of these substances and examines what their actions tell us about the function of these neurotransmitters. A consistent pattern of effects emerges: Norepinephrine underlies the major components of arousal and behaviors that arise in association with increased arousal; dopamine is intimately related to the experience of reward and reward-seeking behaviors. Interestingly, it is also tied into the treatment of—if not directly implicated in the cause of—psychosis.

BASIC NEUROSCIENCE
OF NOREPINEPHRINE AND DOPAMINE

In humans, almost all of the norepinephrine neurons are located within a region called the locus coeruleus (Latin for "blue area") at the base of the brain. The name of this region is related to the fact that these neurons concentrate copper. Although copper is required for the synthesis of norepinephrine, the concentration of the copper far exceeds what is necessary for neurotransmitter synthesis. Unfortunately, the presence of this metal makes these neurons vulnerable to oxygen, which poses a particular risk for the brain. I'll have more to say on this point later in the chapter, but suffice it to say now that the act of breathing oxygen is a mixed blessing for those of us on the planet who have to do it for a living.

The norepinephrine neurons living in your locus coeruleus project throughout your brain. This broad access allows them to influence your level of arousal and thus almost every aspect of your thinking and behavior. Consistent with this role, it has recently been discovered that schizophrenic patients who display a chronic state of hyperarousal have significantly more norepinephrine neurons in their brains.

Although five times more in number than norepinephrine neurons, dopamine neurons do not project as widely throughout your brain. Instead, these neurons, which originate in a region called the midbrain, send projections forward primarily into basal ganglia and frontal lobes. One major dopamine pathway originates within the substantia nigra, or dark substance, so called because this region concentrates the metal iron into a pigmented substance known as melanin. As with the copper in the locus coeruleus, the oxidation of iron (you know this process as rusting) contributes a significant degree of neuronal vulnerability to oxygen. Indeed, many parts of your brain are actually rusting as you breathe. Recent evidence suggests that exposure to common pesticides and insecticides may also accelerate the process of cell death in the substantia nigra. The degeneration of the dopamine neurons in the substantia nigra underlies the progression and symptoms of Parkinson's disease, a disorder characterized by tremors, spasticity, and akinesia, or the absence of movement. These symptoms provide insight into at least one major function of dopamine within your brain. The constant supply of dopamine is necessary to allow you to initiate or inhibit a movement. As you might expect, drugs that interfere with dopamine's normal function (e.g., some antipsychotic medications) produce side effects that resemble those seen in people with Parkinson's disease.

Another pair of dopamine pathways originates in a region of the midbrain near the substantia nigra and ascends upward into the brain. One pathway projects to brain regions that are associated with the control of emotion. The other dopamine pathway projects to the frontal lobes. For more than 50 years, scientists have speculated that excessive activity in these two pathways may underlie some of the symptoms associated with psychosis. We will return to the potential role of dopamine in psychosis later.

The production of dopamine and norepinephrine in your brain begins with the amino acid tyrosine, which is obtained from your diet. Tyrosine is converted to the amino acid levodopa, or L-DOPA, by the enzyme tyrosine hydroxylase. One very important cofactor in this process is iron. Without iron, tyrosine hydroxylase fails to function normally. People with anemia have reduced body levels of iron and, consequently, may have reduced tyrosine hydroxylase activity and thus reduced production of norepinephrine and dopamine. The decreased brain levels of these important neurotransmitters may lead to a slight depression, although most likely only in people with severe anemia. Generally, in a normal healthy person, the production of these two neurotransmitters is not easily affected by the contents of the diet.

Tyrosine can also be acted on by the enzyme tyrosinase and converted into a dark pigment. This enzyme is quite interesting to study because it is vulnerable to a genetic mutation that makes it heat labile (i.e., it only works correctly in the cooler areas of the body). The consequence of this mutation is a lack of pigmentation in humans (albinism) and, conversely, the characteristic pattern of dark pigmentation at the ends of the nose, tail, ears, and paws of Siamese cats (i.e., those parts of the cat that are most distant from their warmer body core). Apparently, this enzyme is critical for the normal decussation, or crossing, of visual tracts, which also underlies the cross-eyed visual problems experienced by Siamese cats. I would suggest that the consequences of this mutation underlie this breed's peculiar personality as well.

The second critical enzymatic step in this pathway is the conversion of L-DOPA into dopamine. This conversion process is extremely efficient, which may explain why brain levels of L-DOPA tend to be very low and why providing exogenous L-DOPA to patients who lack sufficient dopamine— that is, those with Parkinson's disease—leads to a dramatic increase in the production of dopamine. The surviving dopamine neurons in these patients' brains will quickly convert L-DOPA into additional dopamine, which is then released.

There is a third enzyme expressed in norepinephrine neurons that converts dopamine into more norepinephrine; therefore, this enzyme is not expressed by dopamine neurons. The enzyme is stored within the synaptic vesicles and lies in wait for the entry of dopamine molecules once they have been synthesized in the cytoplasm of the neuron. In addition to this third enzyme, the vesicles contain copper and the antioxidant ascorbic acid, also known as vitamin C. Copper is required for the enzyme to function appropriately. The vitamin C maintains the integrity of norepinephrine within the vesicle in the same way that ascorbic acid added to processed meats, such as hotdogs, lengthens the shelf life of these products. Neurons require anti-oxidants such as vitamin C because they are continually exposed to oxygen from the blood. Without vitamin C, many different neurotransmitters oxidize and become inactive while in storage in the vesicles.

All of these energy-demanding enzymatic steps are conducted for the single purpose of ensuring that your vesicles contain an adequate number of biologically active neurotransmitter molecules (usually about 10,000) when they release their contents into the synaptic space between neurons. This is the principal mechanism by which one neuron communicates with the next neuron. What would happen if the vesicles contained no neurotransmitter?

Consider the effects of reserpine, a drug found in the snake root plant (*Rauwolfia serpentina*), which is indigenous to India, Pakistan, Sri Lanka, and Thailand. It prevents the transport of neurotransmitters into the vesicles for storage. If neurotransmitters cannot be stored safely in vesicles, then they are trapped in the cytoplasm, where they will be destroyed. When too many of the vesicles in nerve terminals are empty, it becomes much harder for your neurons to communicate with each other and nervous activity slows down. Therefore, at low doses, reserpine has a tranquilizing effect. At higher doses, because of the greatly reduced availability of these neurotransmitters, reserpine causes severe depression and mood shifts of the sort that might clarify why the snake root plant is called the insanity herb, or "pagla-kadawa," by local Sherpas. The behavioral symptoms are caused by the deficiency of dopamine and norepinephrine, as well as of the neurotransmitter serotonin, and thus offer insight into the role that these neurotransmitters play in the control of arousal and mood. Given this insight, the effects of drugs that enhance the function of dopamine and norepinephrine in your brain should be easy to predict—that is, increased arousal and enhanced mood associated with euphoria. Let's now examine a few of these drugs.

AMPHETAMINES AND ECSTACY

The stimulant drug amphetamine dramatically and rapidly induces the release of norepinephrine and dopamine (and serotonin) into the synapse and greatly slows their inactivation by blocking reuptake back into the neuron. The increased and prolonged presence of these neurotransmitters within the synapse produces heightened alertness, euphoria, lowered fatigue, decreased boredom, depressed appetite, and insomnia. Once amphetamine leaves the brain, the rebound symptoms are extreme fatigue and depression.

During World War II, soldiers and airmen on both sides of the battle lines used amphetamine to combat boredom, fear, and fatigue and to increase endurance. Historians suggest that at end of the war, Adolf Hitler's increasingly paranoid behaviors may have resulted from his excessive use of amphetamines. Indeed, excessive and prolonged use of amphetamine can produce a condition similar to paranoid schizophrenia, and scientists once believed that studying the consequences of high doses

of amphetamine would shed light on the causes of, and potential treatment for, psychosis.

More than half a century later, amphetamines are still popular in the world. However, because of our improved understanding of brain function and advances in medicinal chemistry,
faster-acting and more potent versions of amphetamine have
been invented. How? By making amphetamine more fat-soluble.
One of the basic principles of neuropharmacology is that lipid
(fat) solubility is directly correlated with the speed of uptake of
a drug into the brain. Furthermore, the faster a drug enters the
brain and somehow alters its physiology, the greater the euphoria the drug is likely to induce. This principle has been known
to drug designers for many years. Morphine, for example,
became far more fat soluble and far more euphorigenic (i.e.,
pleasure-inducing) when scientists added two acetyl groups to
it to produce heroin, at the turn of the 19th century. Much later,
amphetamine was similarly modified to make it more euphorigenic and, therefore, more addicting. The simplest manipulation was the addition of a methyl group to make
methamphetamine, a very potent relative of amphetamine that
is far more fat soluble. Not surprisingly, its street name became
"speed" because of its speedy entry into the brain.

Over time, attempts to make amphetamine ever more fat
soluble by the addition of carbon atoms (e.g., in the form of
methyl or ethyl groups) has produced drugs that are more
euphorigenic and hallucinogenic than amphetamine. The most
famous of these is 3,4-methylene-dioxymeth-amphetamine,

widely known as ecstasy. The action of ecstasy in the brain is very similar to amphetamine: It blocks the reuptake of dopamine, norepinephrine, and serotonin and enhances the release of these neurotransmitters. It also produces a dramatic rise in body temperature, or hyperthermia. Indeed, if you were to overdose on ecstasy, hyperthermia would be the cause of your death. How does this happen? Ecstasy has the ability to uncouple the energy-producing capacity of all of the mitochondria in your body. Uncoupling means that mitochondria lose their ability to generate ATP, which is your body's principal energy currency. When they cannot generate ATP, they start wasting their energy as heat. At typical doses of ecstasy, this uncoupling effect is seen most dramatically in the muscles. Because males have more muscle mass than females, on average, males are more sensitive to the acute toxic effects of the hyperthermia.

I have been amazed at the continued popularity of this drug among my students, who seem to believe that because they are young they are also immortal and thus immune to danger. I blame the feelings of immortality on the fact that their frontal lobes are not fully working because they have not yet completed the process of neuronal myelination. Without myelination, electrical signals from neurons fail to reach their destination. The parts of our brains that myelinate last are also the parts that evolved most recently. These parts include our frontal lobes, which contribute most to our unique personalities and allow us to anticipate the consequences of our actions. Essentially, your frontal lobes tell you that it's a bad idea to drink alcohol and drive, or to ignore the consequences of taking ecstasy. When your frontal lobes finally complete their process of myelination, they begin to work properly, and you stop doing stupid things. Most importantly, you stop feeling immortal. Apparently, women finish this process by age 25 years and men finish by age 30. Thus a 20-year-old female, although her brain is still myelinating, is closer to maturity than her 20-year-old boyfriend, who still has another 10 years before he can really hear the sense of warnings such as those against drinking and driving or against taking any drug that comes his way. This delay in brain maturation among males may explain the behavior of many members of college fraternities. But women are not immune. A 19-year-old female student told this story in class one morning: She said that she had met a "nurse" the night before at a bar who offered to give her some pills that she was told would be fun to experience; she only had to return with the "nurse" to her apartment. The characteristics of her experience clearly indicated that the pill contained ecstasy. This young woman did not seem at all disturbed by the fact that she had willingly allowed a total stranger to place her health at risk as a prank. She told us that when she woke in the morning that she just got dressed (?!) and came to class.

MOTHER NATURE'S STIMULANTS

Amphetamine does not occur naturally, but some substances found in nature are chemically related to amphetamine and have similar effects on the brain. Ephedrine can be found in *Ephedra sinica*, which has been used in traditional Chinese medicine and is known as ma huang. Its effects on the sympathetic nervous system are similar to those from amphetamine. However, this extract never achieved complete success as a psychoactive stimulant, primarily because it does not cross the blood–brain barrier as effectively as amphetamine.

Khat is found in an African plant, *Catha edulis*, which contains cathinone and cathine (also known as d-norisoephedrine). The habit of chewing khat to produce a mild arousal probably predates coffee-drinking by centuries. Decoctions, obtained by boiling in hot water, of the khat plant were once known as Abyssinian tea. As is true for most plant-derived biologically active drugs, the relative concentration of khat's active ingredients depends on where the plant is grown, its age, and the time elapsed after it was harvested. Cathinone is quite unstable, a property that makes storage for widespread distribution of the khat plant nearly impossible. You can, of course, purchase dried leaves from this plant in health food stores, but they do not contain any active ingredients. Other compounds in this plant, as in so many others, include chemicals called flavonoids that have anti-inflammatory properties. A few of the 40 different biologically active components of the khat plant also produce the unwanted side effects of green teeth and constipation. Because of the prevalence of this last side effect, the sale of laxatives is quite profitable in countries where khat is widely used.

Another naturally occurring drug that is similar to amphet-amine can be found in the cactus *Lophophora williamsii*. Extracts are used to prepare a drink called peyote that contains 3,4,5-trimethoxyphenyl-ethylamine (the "meth" and "phenyl" point to a molecule that is quite fat soluble). Known as mescaline, this compound is structurally similar to the catechol-amines dopamine and norepinephrine but seems to act more directly on serotonin receptors because of the presence of the methoxy groups on the molecule. This feature of the compound's structure would make the compound more fat soluble and therefore better able to enter the brain quickly and may explain why mescaline produces an amphetamine-like euphoria at low doses and hallucinations at higher doses. Indeed, this euphoria-to-hallucination transition is a common dose-dependent characteristic of many psychoactive plant extracts.

Mescaline is either poorly metabolized or not metabolized at all by humans. Therefore, various and rather rigid cultural rituals developed a "recycling" program for the experience of ingesting it. Often, persons of highest social or religious rank would consume mescaline in large quantities, eventually passing it in their urine, which was then consumed by those of lesser social status. Sometimes, because of the gradual loss of potency, the urine from a few people needed to be combined to achieve the greatly anticipated experience. The Vikings were thus not the only group of ancient peoples willing to drink someone else's urine for a good time.

This reminds me of one of my students, a young woman, who claimed that her boyfriend liked to cook sections of this cactus into a lasagna-like preparation that he layered with ricotta cheese and tomatoes. She was curious whether the mescaline in his urine would remain active if she saved the urine for later use. Once you get past the obvious concerns about the sterility and purity of the collected urine (and the disturbing mental imagery), the active ingredient would probably be quite stable if stored frozen in orange or grapefruit juice to lower the pH of the urine. This approach would, as she observed, avoid the nasty gastrointestinal side effects that usually accompany eating this cactus because of the presence of nonpsychoactive compounds that affect the gut's dopamine and serotonin neurons.

The drug asarone, which comes from a plant, *Acorus calamus* (found in Asia, Europe, and North America), is chemically very similar to mescaline. The roots of this plant are chewed to produce a dose-dependent effect; about 2 inches of the root produces a mild euphoria, whereas nearly 10 inches produces hallucinations. In some cultures, wives will chew on the roots and collect their saliva throughout the day for their husbands to enjoy later. Nothing says "welcome home" at the end of a hard day like a nice warm bowl of spit.

Various psychoactive spices have also been discovered that alter the function of the brain's dopamine, norepinephrine, and serotonin neurons. For example, the spice nutmeg comes from the nutmeg tree, *Myristica fragrans*, and contains myristicin, which is also chemically quite similar to mescaline. (Myristicin is found in parsley and carrots as well but at very low concentrations.) Typically, one must consume about 30 grams of nutmeg powder—or roughly the contents of an entire container of the product you could purchase at your local grocery store—to experience its psychoactive effects. Reactions vary considerably, from nothing at all, to euphoria at low doses, to marijuana- and D-lysergic acid diethylamide (LSD)–like experiences at higher doses, with hallucinations that can last up to 48 hours. Chronic use of high doses of nutmeg can produce a reaction similar to psychosis. One other unpleasant side effect of nutmeg is extreme diarrhea caused by the stimulation of dopamine and serotonin neurons within the gut. It has been claimed to be an aphrodisiac. Perhaps for that reason, one of my students consumed an entire canister of nutmeg that he had dissolved in some applesauce; the weekend he spent in the bathroom demonstrated why most people never try nutmeg more than once.

Spices such as saffron, fennel, dill, cinnamon, and anise also contain psychoactive substances that are chemically similar to myristicin. Generally, the level of psychoactive agents in these other spices is far too low to produce any noticeable consequences in people using them for cooking, but their role, regardless of how subtle, in enhancing the culinary experience should not be ignored.

Similar amphetamine-like substances have been found in kava kava, a drink prepared from roots of a pepper tree, *Piper methysticum*, which grows in the South Pacific islands. *Piper* is Latin for "pepper"; *methysticum* is Greek for "intoxicating." The drink contains various potentially psychoactive resins that include kawain and methysticin. As is true for the complex ingredients of most plants, the psychoactive efficacy of the kava extract does not arise from any one of these compounds but rather from a blending of their effects in the brain. These resins are capable of stimulating dopamine and GABA receptors, and so their actions are similar to the effects of amphetamine and to those of some popular antianxiety drugs. The resins from this plant are quite fat soluble and thus will enter the brain relatively easily and quickly to produce a relaxed euphoria and sometimes, at high doses, hallucinations.

Half a coconut shell (the typical way it's consumed) will contain approximately 150 milliliters of a foul-tasting, muddy liquid. Sometimes the kava preparation is strong enough to put a drinker into a deep, dreamless sleep within 30 minutes. One of my students tried it and reported the hallucination as follows: "The top of my head just blew off!" Not an appealing mental image. Fresh kava kava rootstock yields a greenish milky solution that is considerably stronger than the grayer mixture obtained from dry roots.

It is possible to go into many upscale grocery stores and purchase extracts of kava kava plants, but their ingredients are no longer active. Real kava kava tends to be unstable, particularly with the liquid storage that is commonly used in these products. Given the unstable nature of the ingredients of this plant, the presumed antianxiety actions of kava kava extracts obtained in U.S. stores results entirely from the placebo effect.

COCAINE

The comedian Robin Williams once quipped that cocaine is God's way of telling you that you're making too much money. The United States must indeed be a wealthy country, considering that 3 million of our fellow citizens abuse this drug; this is six times the number of heroin addicts in our nation. It is estimated that 50% of Americans between the ages of 25 and 30 years have tried cocaine.

What does cocaine do in the brain? First, it binds to sodium ion channels and blocks them from functioning. This action stops the flow of action potentials and prevents neurons from communicating with each other. Cocaine also blocks the conduction of pain signals, which explains why, after it was isolated from the coca plant (*Erythroxylon coca*) in 1855, it was used as a local anesthetic, including for the eye and for toothaches. But ultimately, its anesthetic actions would be discovered to have nothing to do with the reason for its later illegal street use: its ability to produce euphoria.

Cocaine acts similarly to amphetamine with regard to its ability to enhance the effects of dopamine and serotonin at the synapse. The actions of cocaine on the brain lead to increased alertness, reduced hunger, increased physical and mental endurance, increased motor activity, and an intensification of most normal pleasures. This last feature may explain why so many claim that cocaine enhances emotional and sexual feelings. Cocaine abusers usually co-administer other drugs that are brain depressants (e.g., alcohol, heroin, or marijuana) to decrease the unpleasant hyperstimulant aspects of cocaine.

Approximately 16 to 32 milligrams of cocaine is an effective street dosage that is usually without immediate negative side effects. An increase in heart rate usually occurs within about 8 minutes after administration and dissipates 30 to 40 minutes later. The half-life, or the time it takes for half of the drug to exit the blood and body, is about 40 to 50 minutes. Cocaine will actually degrade spontaneously in the body to produce an inactive compound with a tongue-twister name, benzoylecgonine. The physiological effects of cocaine are therefore much shorter than those of amphetamine. Partly for this reason, most users claim that it does not "wear out" the body in the same way that amphetamine does.

Getting cocaine to its site of action within the brain first requires getting adequate amounts of the drug into the blood. Snuffing cocaine by applying it to mucous membranes inside the nose is much more effective than either oral administration or intravenous use, because the drug enters the blood and brain more quickly and is therefore more immediately euphorigenic. Unfortunately, there is a problem with this approach to getting cocaine into the blood. Cocaine constricts the blood vessels feeding the cartilage in the bridge of the nose and, with repeated nasal application, leads to the ischemic (lack of blood) death of the tissues supporting the end of the nose. Initially, the irritation to the tissue causes a runny nose; ultimately, the irritation leads to a true necrosis, or cell death, and the end of the nose either collapses or becomes quite distorted.

Orally administered cocaine is not well absorbed from the gastrointestinal tract, and its effects on the brain thus tend to be far less reinforcing when taken in this fashion. But oral administration does have a long history. Many years before cocaine extracts were applied to mucous membranes, ancient peoples simply ate the leaves of the coca plant. Indeed, although cocaine use peaked in the 1880s and the 1980s, chewing coca leaves for their psychoactive effects—they contain up to 1% of cocaine by weight—was a popular practice long before these eras. The leaves have been found in 5,000-year-old graves. Approximately 800 years ago in South America, people started chewing the leaves wrapped around a piece of limestone to increase the pH in their mouths and to augment the release of cocaine from the leaves. By improving the extraction of cocaine from the leaves, the experience became far more pleasurable. The Incas introduced religious ritual to its use and invented the word "cocata" to describe the distance a person could walk on one chew of coca leaf before the beneficial effects wore off. The tribal chiefs gave coca leaves to runners in the Andes Mountains to help them tolerate the altitude and to increase their endurance; the runners were also paid in coca leaves, thus maintaining their addiction and continued service until they died of exhaustion and malnutrition. The conquering Spanish subsequently recognized the cost-saving wisdom in this approach and paid their Incan servants with coca leaves, enabling them to work harder and eat less food. Amerigo Vespucci, who gave his name to the newly "discovered" land, wrote about the use of coca leaves by the local tribes.

Fast-forward a number of centuries, and we see the oral use of coca plant extracts taking a new form. In 1862, Angelo Mariani, a Corsican chemist, combined a Bordeaux wine with coca plant extracts to produce and sell "Vin Mariani." The labels displayed testimonials from Pope Leo XIII, who gave it the Vatican's gold medal of appreciation, as well as from President Ulysses S. Grant and from Thomas Edison, who claimed that it helped him stay awake longer to complete his experiments. Vin Mariani was such a commercial success that many other alcohol-based tonics containing coca leaf extracts were introduced in the late 1880s. One quite successful tonic was introduced by John S. Pemberton in 1884. Pemberton called his drink "a French wine of coca, ideal tonic." Later, in 1886, he removed the alcohol, replaced cocaine with an extract from the kola nut, and called it Coca-Cola. But why combine coca leaf extracts with wine in the first place? The reason is that the combined effect of these two drugs on the brain is far more euphorigenic, and therefore more addicting, than either compound alone. When combined with alcohol, as in Vin Mariani, the mixture forms a powerful psychoactive compound called coca-ethylene, which is more fat soluble than cocaine and thus enters the brain faster; by now you know what that implies in terms of the enhanced pleasure it will produce.

Drug designers are never far behind the chemists in discovering new ways to make drugs enter the brain faster. After all, greater addiction of one's customers leads to higher profits. Thus, in the 1960s, free-base cocaine was produced and people discovered that it very quickly entered the blood and brain and produced an ever greater euphoria. The natural product that had been obtained from the coca leaf for so many centuries exists as cocaine hydrochloride; this is an acidic compound that can be volatilized—that is, turned into a vapor. However, at a high temperature, the cocaine is destroyed. This is why naturally occurring cocaine was never smoked; the active ingredient is completely lost. I would predict that someone somewhere at some time must have tried smoking coca leaves and found that it was a disappointing failure. To be effective when smoked, cocaine must be reconverted chemically to its alkaloid, or base, form. The process of converting and then isolating the product is called free-basing. The conversion process requires the use of highly flammable solvents that, when not properly handled, can set celebrities (e.g., the comedian Richard Pryor) and other people on fire.

More recently, modifications in the process of making the basic form of the drug have produced cocaine crystals that spontaneously generate small chunks; this product is called crack—related to the sound the crystals make when heated. It can be smoked and, therefore, will deliver cocaine into the brain as fast as an intravenous injection, but without the inconvenient and potentially unhealthy process of using a needle.

Cocaine is so rewarding that its users prefer it to sex, food, and water, thus overriding basic survival drives. In experiments, laboratory animals will self-administer cocaine to the point of severe toxicity, physical exhaustion, and even death. Many human users support their habit by selling cocaine or by stealing from friends and coworkers. Even Sigmund Freud, who wrote a scholarly and quite accurate treatise on cocaine's effects, in "Über Coca" (1884), got carried away and claimed his use of the drug cured his morphine addiction. In fact, it simply became a second addiction for him.

The compelling and overwhelming nature of cocaine addiction is impressive and tells us something profound about how the brain is built. It is apparently comprised of critically important internal neural systems that can produce a powerful rewarding experience usually connected to activities that are the basis for the survival of our species: eating and reproduction. Drugs such as cocaine can hijack these neural processes and stimulate the brain's reward centers so excessively and unnaturally that users will crave more stimulation, as they would normally crave food and sex. From the brain's perspective, there is no real difference between these cravings. Thus, the familiar moral fiber argument of "just say no" is unbelievably naïve, and its application cruel. It ignores the complexities of the brain and the influence of culture and evolution on how the brain responds to drugs.

How precisely does cocaine achieve these effects in the brain? As described in Chapter 1, once a neurotransmitter is released from its neuronal terminal, its actions within the synapse are ended principally by reuptake into the presynaptic terminal. Cocaine primarily blocks the reuptake of dopamine but also acts similarly on norepinephrine and serotonin reuptake. If your neuronal terminals can be seen as acting like little vacuum cleaners, then cocaine essentially clogs the vacuum nozzle. As a consequence of this blockade, the concentrations of dopamine, norepinephrine, and serotonin within the synaptic cleft between two neurons increase dramatically. Within millions of synapses in the brain, these neurotransmitters are now free to continue to stimulate their receptors over and over, again and again. There are neuronal terminals for dopamine, norepinephrine, and serotonin scattered throughout the entire brain, and thus the consequences of cocaine on brain function are also widespread.

And as we have seen before, what happens after a drug exits the brain tells us something about what parts of the brain were affected under the influence of that drug. With regard to cocaine, these include the arousal systems within the brainstem, the feeding centers within the hypothalamus, and the reward centers within the frontal lobes and limbic system. Thus, cocaine reduces the need for sleep, and its absence produces extreme sleepiness; it reduces the desire to eat, and its absence is associated with increased food consumption; it produces extreme euphoria, and its absence leads to a severe depression (it is thought that the emotional highs and lows that cocaine abuse produces over time may explain the origin of the novella, *The Strange Case of Dr. Jekyll and Mr. Hyde,* by Robert Louis Stevenson). Excessive, long-term, intravenous use of cocaine tends to produce especially severe rebound phenomena, including psychotic behaviors together with delusions of grandeur and hallucinations. For many drugs that affect the brain, including cocaine, the degree of rebound symptoms is typically related to how many times a person has used the drug. Moreover, the effects of cocaine on brain chemistry and physiology may be long term. Even after withdrawal from the drug, most chronic users report visual disturbances such as "snow lights" and other sensory disturbances such as formication, or the feeling of bugs crawling on the skin; these symptoms usually only occur after prolonged use of cocaine. These delayed effects might be viewed as echoes of neural activity reverberating within the circuits of the brain following the powerful stimulation produced by the cocaine.

Lidocaine is chemically similar to cocaine; it is also a sodium channel–blocking drug, which is why it is an effective topical pain reliever commonly sold over the counter in drug stores. However, in contrast to cocaine, it has no reinforcing, euphoric effect at all, and animals, including humans, will not self-administer it. This confirms the validity of the finding that the anesthetic actions of cocaine do not contribute to its ability to produce euphoria.

But what explains why we experience euphoria from cocaine or amphetamine or ecstasy? Euphoria is the brain's unfailing response to the fast entry of drugs that increase the level of the neurotransmitter dopamine in the synapse between neurons. Again, increasing the fat solubility of these drugs speeds their entry into the brain and makes them more pleasurable. The brain behaves as though it likes drugs that quickly change its level of activity. Just how does dopamine facilitate this experience?

DOPAMINE: THE GAS PEDAL
OF PLEASURE

Much of our current evidence provides only indirect confirmation of dopamine's role in experiencing pleasure. First, every drug of abuse somehow enhances the function of dopamine neurons. Probably everything we choose to do for pleasure, including eating or having sex or listening to beautiful music, somehow affects our dopamine neurons. Second, drugs that antagonize the function of dopamine, such as the antipsychotic drugs discussed in the next section, greatly reduce our ability to experience pleasure. Third, dopamine sets the pace at which the frontal lobes process information, akin to setting the ticking rate of a clock. The faster your clock ticks, the faster your brain processes information. Drugs that increase the release of dopamine often speed up your thinking process. They also produce increased motor activity, such as pacing and fidgeting. We see these side effects in children treated with drugs, all of which are chemically modified molecules of amphetamine, for attention-deficit/hyperactivity disorder; their performance in school improves but they are more hyperactive. Drugs such as amphetamine and cocaine speed up the clock, whereas drugs that impair the function of dopamine, such as the antipsychotics, tend to slow mental processing speed. With normal aging, the slow decline in the release of dopamine in the frontal lobes gradually slows one's ability to process information as quickly as one could when younger. Patients with Parkinson's disease, caused by the degeneration of dopamine neurons, suffer from the slowing of their higher cognitive abilities and from emotional depression, including the inability to experience pleasure. The drugs that patients with Parkinson's take to lessen their symptoms enhance the function of dopamine and tend to produce a slight euphoria and, occasionally, an increase in the incidence of compulsive behaviors, such as gambling.

Considered together, the effects of a diverse array of drugs all signify that your brain is a race car and that dopamine is the gas pedal. Your brain "feels" euphoria when the gas pedal is pushed quickly (by ever-increasing fat solubility), and your thoughts are allowed to fly as fast as possible around your mental track. The forces of evolution have shaped your brain to truly enjoy working fast—the faster the better because fast brains are more likely to exist within creatures who survive and who will therefore pass on this trait to the next generation. Thus, classic Darwinism underlies why we enjoy what we enjoy so much, be it having sex, or eating chocolate, or ingesting drugs of abuse like amphetamine, ecstasy, and cocaine.

TREATING PSYCHOSIS

What happens when the gas pedal is stuck full on? Is this the basis of psychosis? What can be done to fix it? Whatever the causes of psychosis may be, almost universally, the treatment is to block dopamine receptors. Most of the catecholamine-enhancing drugs that I've discussed thus far interfere with the ability of the brain's presynaptic neurons to produce, store, and release or inactivate the neurotransmitters dopamine and nor-epinephrine. Antipsychotic drugs, however, work at the other side of the synapse, achieving considerable therapeutic efficacy in many psychotic patients by blocking the function of their dopamine receptors in postsynaptic neurons. Let's look at what this action can teach us about the function of dopamine in the brain and the neurological mechanisms underlying psychosis.

Psychosis is essentially a generic term for a mental condition associated with a loss of contact with reality. Individuals who are psychotic report hallucinations, delusions, and highly disorganized thinking. As a result, they tend to have great difficulty functioning in their daily lives and have trouble sustaining normal social interactions with others. Drugs that block dopamine receptors are capable of reducing some of the symptoms associated with psychosis. But herein lies a complexity: In no way do the antipsychotic effects of these drugs prove that psychosis is caused by a dysfunction of dopamine neurons, any more than reducing depressive symptoms in some people through medications that selectively block reuptake of dopamine, norepinephrine, or serotonin proves that a dysfunction of these neurotransmitters underlies depression. This is a very important general point to consider when examining drug action as a way of understanding brain function.

In fact, an alteration in dopamine function probably does not cause psychosis; rather, it is most likely just a secondary consequence of a complex array of alterations of one or more different neural systems in the brain. This may explain why the blockade of some dopamine receptors within certain brain regions reduces the severity of a few bothersome psychotic symptoms but not others. The antagonism of dopamine receptors may simply compensate for the presence of an error of chemistry that exists somewhere in the brain. Whatever the reason for their efficacy, all we know for certain is that antipsychotics that block dopamine receptors provide significant benefits for some, but not all, patients.

Unfortunately, these drugs—especially the "first generation" of antipsychotics introduced in the 1950s—have side effects similar to those seen in patients with Parkinson's disease: tremors when at rest, reduction of voluntary movement, muscle spasticity and dystonia, or sustained muscle contractions. These symptoms confirm the role of dopamine neurons in the initiation and control of movement. Antipsychotic drugs also block dopamine receptors within a region of the brain that controls the release of the hormone prolactin. The result is an increase in the release of prolactin and thus an increase in breast tissue growth. Increased breast development can be very disturbing to male patients who may already be paranoid about the medications they are prescribed.

Newer, "second-generation" antipsychotics have side effects as well—for example, they may cause significant weight gain that many patients find frustrating. Recent evidence suggests that the weight gain is related to the blockade of histamine receptors in the brain. Interestingly, the original clinical use of the first antipsychotic drug, chlorpromazine (sold as Thorazine in the United States), occurred because of its ability to block histamine receptors and reduce symptoms of the common cold; only later was it recognized that this drug could also reduce psychotic symptoms. Recently, the connection between histamine and dopamine in the brain became even more interesting. Apparently, many of the newer over-the-counter antihistamine medications are capable of blocking the reuptake of dopamine in a manner reminiscent of cocaine. Suddenly, treating one's sniffles has become a far more euphorigenic experience!

In a manner similar to that observed following treatment with antidepressant drugs, the side effects of dopamine receptor blockade occur rather quickly, but the clinical benefits require 2 to 3 weeks, or more, to fully develop. This also implies that compensatory changes in brain function are required for these drugs to produce clinical benefits in psychotic patients. These changes most likely require the activation or inactivation of genes in a specific population of neurons within selected brain regions.

By now you have a sense of the interwoven roles of dopamine, norepinephrine, and acetylcholine in the control of movement, reward, mood, arousal, and learning and attention. By considering how various drugs manipulate these neurotransmitter systems within the brain, scientists have discovered some consistent patterns that allow us to make predictions about what to expect when specific types of drugs are taken. The same holds true for the neurotransmitter system mentioned several times in this chapter: serotonin. What are the consequences of its manipulation in the brain? Read on.

CHAPTER 5

Your Brain's Anchor to Reality

How does the brain filter incoming sensory information so that sights and sounds do not become all mixed together? What happens when the brain loses this filtering ability as a result of, say, taking a hallucinogenic drug? What have we learned about depression and anxiety from the drugs that we administer to treat these disorders? The answers to these questions are slowly being revealed as more becomes known about the actions of serotonin in the brain.

Serotonin is a very ancient neurotransmitter and has been found in the venom of amphibians, wasps, and scorpions and within the nematocysts of the sea anemone as well as in the nervous system of parasitic flatworms, crickets, and lobsters. Within the human body, 90% of the total serotonin is contained within the neurons of the gut and is released from the intestines to determine bone growth or shrinkage. Another 8% of the body's serotonin is found in the blood and is localized inside platelets and mast cells; in fact, it was initially discovered in serum and determined to have tonic (or constricting) effects on the vascular system—hence its name. The remaining few percent is found in the brain, in roughly the same location as in every other vertebrate brain, leading scientists to conclude that this neurotransmitter system was present in the primitive nervous system at least one-half billion years ago.

THE POWER OF A FEW PERCENT

Neurons that produce and release serotonin in the brain are organized into a series of nuclei that lie in a chain along the midline, or seam, of the brainstem; these are called the raphe nuclei (*raphe* means "seam" in Latin). These neurons project their axons to every part of the brain, and some of these axons make contact with blood vessels; the neurons also project downward into the spinal cord. If you were able to insert a recording device into the major raphe nuclei and "listen" to the activity of your serotonin neurons, you would discover that they have a regular, slow spontaneous level of activity that varies little while you are awake. When you fall asleep, the activity of these neurons slows. When you start to dream—or if, as we'll see shortly, you ingest a hallucinogen—these neurons cease their activity completely.

Despite the relative scarcity of serotonin in your brain, drugs that alter serotonin function can produce profound changes in how you feel and how you experience the world around you. For example, such drugs often stimulate the sympathetic autonomic nervous system and produce increased heart rate, increased respiration, dilated pupils, and other unpleasant side effects. On the other hand, the effects of serotonin on blood vessel dilation may underlie the ability of an entire class of drugs, known as the triptans, to attenuate the pain associated with a migraine headache. Other drugs can also help alleviate symptoms that often accompany migraines and that involve serotonin: depression and sleep problems.

The production of serotonin requires the absorption of the amino acid tryptophan from your food. Transport of this amino acid is influenced by the level of other amino acids in your blood; that level, in turn, is also influenced by what you eat. Within the neurons of your brain, tryptophan is converted to 5-hydroxy-tryptophan by tryptophan hydroxylase. This enzyme is never completely inundated with tryptophan—mainly because it is so challenging for tryptophan to be transported across the blood–brain barrier. Therefore, if you eat less tryptophan, your brain generally produces less serotonin. Studies have shown that consuming a diet low in tryptophan can negatively influence serotonin-controlled brain processes that affect emotion and sleep.

Can dietary supplements increase brain tryptophan levels and improve mood? The answer is no. There is no evidence for improving mood through dietary manipulation of tryptophan, primarily because it is difficult to change plasma tryptophan levels through diet alone. Tryptophan supplementation and depletion studies suggest that altering tryptophan levels may only affect certain groups of patients who have a personal or family history of depression. Popular media articles often recommend diets and foods to increase blood tryptophan levels and raise brain serotonin levels. Such recommendations, while superficially appealing, are misleading and not supported by any current scientific studies.

Moreover, the release of serotonin from neurons in the brain can be prevented, and this has been correlated with the initiation of hallucinations. This is not to say that we can manipulate our diet to undermine serotonin release so as to experience a hallucination. We cannot. But certain drugs that will initiate this effect, and their action, as well as the experiences they produce, can tell us something about the normal function of serotonin in the brain.

HALLUCINOGENS

How do hallucinogens work? One hallucinogenic drug, LSD, binds to a variety of different serotonin-sensitive receptors on the surface of neurons; initially, LSD slows their rate of firing. At the left side of Figure 5.1, you can see graphically what the activity of serotonin would look like if you placed an electrode into one of the raphe nuclei in the brainstem and then administered LSD to it. At first, the firing is quite regular. The arrow in the figure shows when LSD was injected into the brain. Only a few minutes later, you can see that the activity of the serotonin neurons slows way down, similar to that seen when we enter dream sleep. But that similarity is only a neat coincidence; the half-life of LSD is about 3 hours, at which time the hallucinatory effects reach their peak—but studies using radioactively labeled LSD have shown that at this time there are no detectable LSD molecules in the brain! The psychoactive effect of LSD far outlasts the slowing of serotonin neural activity; therefore, the slowed activity of serotonin neurons does not explain why we hallucinate on this drug and why the hallucinations are so similar to dreaming. Indeed, the effects of LSD on serotonin neurons may only be the initial trigger that sets in motion a cascade of complex processes throughout the brain that is experienced as a hallucination.

A naturally occurring version of LSD is D Lysergic acid monoethylamide. It is slightly less fat soluble (one less ethyl group) than LSD, but it too can produce hallucinations. *Claviceps*

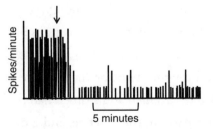

Figure 5.1. The activity of serotonin would look like this if you placed an electrode into one of the raphe nuclei in the brainstem. If LSD is administered at the arrow, then the activity of these cells slows down.

purpurea, the ergot fungus that produces this compound, also generates a toxin that mimics the action of serotonin, particularly its ability to constrict blood vessels. Consumption of bread made from grain or corn that is contaminated with this fungus causes a burning in the extremities resulting from extreme constriction of blood vessels and leads to limb death. One outbreak of ergotism, as this condition came to be known, may have caused the death of nearly 40,000 people in Europe in 944 CE; at that time, it was called *ignis sacer,* or "Saint Anthony's holy fire," after the monks of the Order of St. Anthony. Consumption of ergot-contaminated grains may also have been responsible for a number of mystical experiences reported in the past, including those that took place annually during the ancient Greek ceremonies known as the Eleusinian Mysteries. Some historians even believe that ergot-contaminated rye may have caused the behaviors that eventually led to the Salem witchcraft trials that began in December of 1691. According to available records, eight girls suffered with "distempers" that included, according to witnesses, "disorderly speech, odd postures and gestures, and convulsive fits." Although ergotism was quite familiar to medical science and to historians by the 17th century, the New England Puritans chose to see these symptoms as the work of Satan brought about by the practice of witchcraft. By September of 1692, 20 men and women had been tried and executed for "their part" in the practice, and 2 died in prison.

Psilocybin, a chemically similar naturally occurring molecule, is much less potent than LSD but likely shares aspects of its actions on serotonin neurons once the body converts it into psilocin. Our ancestors probably discovered its sources, *Psilocybe mexicana, P. semilanceata,* and *P. cyanescens,* by accident when foraging for edible mushrooms. Just imagine how horrific and unexpected the experience must have been for the first person who inadvertently prepared one of these mushrooms for consumption, bringing new meaning to the phrase "dinner and a show."

Sixteenth-century Central American Indians, according to the naturalist Francisco Hernandez, called these mushrooms "Teonanácatl," possibly translated as "God's flesh" or, simply, "sacred mushroom." Albert Hofmann, the scientist credited with the inadvertent discovery of LSD when investigating its effects, is also credited with isolating the active ingredient of this mushroom, in 1958. He claimed to have ingested 32 dried mushrooms, probably 10 times the usual dose taken today, to determine their effects and wrote that they were similar to those he had experienced with LSD. It's worth stating the obvious at this point—please do not ever experiment with unknown plant extracts on yourself, especially if there is any risk that they might affect your brain. I know this warning seems self-evident, but I've had too many students bring empty vials to my class saying: "I took this last night and I was wondering if you could tell me what it was?" These questions might actually seem appropriate when you're 19 years old and feel immortal.

Psilocybin can, in fact, be found in more than 75 different species of mushrooms. It is also chemically similar to bufotenine, an interesting hallucinogenic molecule that is chemically very similar in structure to serotonin. Bufotenine has been discovered in a truly diverse set of locations: the skin and glands of a South American toad, seed pods from the South American tree, *Piptadenia peregrina*, and the leaves and bark of the Central American mimosa, *Acacia niopo*. The seeds from *Piptadenia peregrina* are ground with limestone to increase the extraction of the bufotenine, much as tobacco companies today add ammonia to raise the pH and increase the absorption of nicotine in your mouth. The grounded blend of bean pod and limestone is used as a snuff called "yopo." Young boys blow the snuff into each other's nostrils through a forked tube made from hollow chicken bones. Interestingly, bufotenine may also be present in the *Amanita muscaria* mushroom, which may be responsible for some of the psychoactive effects described in Chapter 4. The actions of bufotenine on the brain are still speculative because no one has yet demonstrated that it can actually cross the blood–brain barrier. Bufotenine's reputation may be more directly related to its toxic effects outside of the brain.

In fact, no one is currently certain how LSD or any of the hallucinogens actually works, or just how serotonin factors into their hallucinatory effects. Confounding this uncertainty is the fact that some hallucinogens have no apparent effect on serotonin at all. For example, salvinorin A, from the Mexican plant *Salvia divinorum*, is a very potent naturally occurring hallucinogenic compound that is similar to morphine in its actions but has no identified action at serotonin receptors.

WHAT ARE HALLUCINATIONS?

The complex sensory experiences known as hallucinations can, however, occur from other sources besides drugs like LSD or psilocybin, and this fact may shed some light on the nature of the hallucinatory experience, drug-induced or otherwise, and its connection to serotonin. Consider, for example, the following hypothetical scenario:

Imagine yourself as a newborn lying in a crib. Your brain's serotonin neurons at this age, and during the first couple years of your life, are not working completely because the neurons and glia that support them have not fully developed. In addition, the makeup of serotonin receptors at this age has not yet converted to the adult balance of excitatory and inhibitory subtypes of receptors. Your sensory systems—visual, auditory, and olfactory abilities in particular—are working, but your serotonergic system is not adequately installed to assist them with the processing of the incoming sensory information to the brain. Suddenly, you sense something looming over your crib—a large green, distorted face with a screeching voice and reeking of a yellow odor—and you scream in fear. You have just had your first hallucination. You have also just experienced synesthesia, or the merging and mixing of sensory processes—for example, sights that produce sounds or smells that have color.

Now imagine yourself 20 years later, with your serotonergic system fully developed. Let's assume that you yourself are not actually a "synesthete," that rare person who has this condition that mixes data from the different senses as an inherited part of his or her life. But take a hallucinogenic drug at age 20 years (or any adult age), and you could have a temporary synesthetic experience similar to what you had in your crib as an infant. Why? The inhibited function of your serotonergic system that is induced by a hallucinogen may reproduce the condition of synesthesia that was simply "normal" when you were a newborn. As a newborn, you would find this condition to be frightening. But as an adult who has taken a hallucinogen, you might, in the right setting, come to believe that the condition is a transcendently mystical experience.

SEROTONIN AND RELIGIOSITY

Timothy Leary, the famous LSD guru of the 1960s counterculture movement, once commented in 1964, "A psychedelic experience is a journey to new realms of consciousness. The scope and content of the experience is limitless, but its characteristic features are the transcendence of verbal concepts, of space time dimensions, and of the ego and identity." His description has a spiritual flavor that might be very familiar to people who are skillful at tantric yoga or transcendental meditation. Mind-altering or mind-expanding drugs, usually referring to hallucinogens, alter your consciousness, your sense of personal space and time, and your perception of the real world around you. In reality, the actions of hallucinogens in the brain that lead to an "expanding of the mind" probably result from relatively subtle alterations in normal serotonin neuronal function.

These changes, as I mentioned earlier, set in motion a cascade of poorly understood neural processes that impair aspects of normal consciousness.

One function of consciousness, and a role probably influenced by serotonin, is its ability to filter out the overwhelming and confusing mass of sensory input that your brain receives while you are awake. If you lose the ability to filter incoming sensory stimuli, you would probably become very disoriented and confused. Drug-induced mind expansion can therefore only be experienced safely—that is, so as to avoid completely freaking out—in a highly structured and protected setting. It should come as no surprise then that many cultures have developed strict religious and social rules around the use of plants that produce hallucinations. Extracts from psychoactive plants, or symbolic representations of them such as the burning of incense, have often played a significant role in religious ceremonies. Indeed, the near-universal co-occurrence of religion and the use of natural hallucinatory agents may point to the crossroads that connect various hypotheses on why religiosity is so common across diverse primitive societies.

What I am suggesting is that the appearance of the small mystical societies in ancient times that ultimately evolved into more familiar organized religions was assisted by the near-universal presence of hallucinogenic plants that were able to alter how the brain functioned and to facilitate each culture's communication with their gods and goddesses. If true, then it should also come as no surprise that in recorded history, humans have worshiped more than 2,500 major deities; the actual number is probably far greater. The similarities between a hallucinatory experience and, for some, an intense religious experience are consistent with the hypothesis that religion has a biological basis that was shaped by our shared evolution with, and constant exposure to, the hallucinatory plants around us. The widespread use of hallucinogenic plants by our ancestors may underlie some of the fantastic stories that have become associated with various religions. For example, some people believe that the first chapter of the Book of Ezekiel describes this prophet's encounter with beings from outer space during the sixth century BCE; a more reasonable explanation might be that the experience was initiated by the consumption of an hallucinogenic plant targeting the brain's serotonergic system. Therefore, because serotonin neurons play a role in how hallucinogens interact with the brain, it is also possible that serotonin plays a role in the individual expressions of religiosity across cultures.

In addition, there may be a correlation between religiosity, specific genetic markers underlying the function of serotonin, and other mental experiences besides hallucinations. Genetically altered mice and positron emission tomography (PET) studies on humans have been very useful in demonstrating the potential role of specific serotonin receptors in the regulation of mood and anxiety. For example, mice lacking a particular serotonin receptor, known as type 5HT-1A, show more anxiety-like behavior. Some recently discovered drugs target this receptor to reduce the symptoms of depression and anxiety in humans. The overall effectiveness of these drugs at least suggests that this receptor in particular may play an important role in the normal control of anxiety or mood.

So what is the connection to one's personal degree of religiosity? The number of type 5HT-1A serotonin receptors in the brain is inversely correlated with self-ratings of religiosity and spirituality. People who respond negatively (e.g., with excessive anxiety or depression) to the challenges of everyday life have fewer 5HT-1A receptors and are more likely to find comfort in religious faith and practice. Moreover, a series of studies have demonstrated that people with certain serotonin receptor profiles suffer more often with social anxiety disorder, which is characterized by an extreme fear that other people are thinking bad things about them. Fortunately, these people also tend to respond more positively to placebos or affirmative suggestions than people who do not have these types of serotonin receptors in their brain. Taken together, these findings suggest that people who yearn for more religious leadership in their lives may have inherited fewer serotonin receptors than those who never express such yearnings.

Before drawing too close of a correlation between religiosity and the number of type-1A serotonin receptors, we should recognize that other features of the brain also correlate with the tendency to rate oneself as religious. A recent investigation discovered that the tendency to display extravagant religious behaviors correlated significantly with atrophy (i.e., shrinkage) of the right hippocampus in patients with untreatable epilepsy. In fact, the medical literature is replete with reports of epilepsy patients with religious delusions. Decreased brain activity in the hippocampus has also been correlated with the feeling of a "sensed presence" or the eerie feeling of an unseen person nearby. Recent studies using sophisticated brain imaging techniques also suggest that the prefrontal cortex is more likely involved in controlling our religious, moral, and paranormal beliefs.

To understand why the brain generates religious sensations under these unusual conditions, it is necessary to appreciate what it does under normal circumstances. Usually, your brain receives sensory inputs from your body and produces a sense of where you are in the world, what you are doing at this moment, and what is happening all around you. This incoming information is constantly updated and provides you with a sense of "self." If your senses are impaired or your brain's ability to interpret sensory information is altered because of an hallucinogenic drug or a disorder like epilepsy, your brain is forced to do the best it can with what it has working. Thus, under these conditions, you might have some very unusual sensory experiences, such as feelings of floating in space, a connection to everything in the universe, or a communication with your god, however you might see him or her.

You can clearly see that, for lack of any more precise way to quantify these experiences, neuroscientists often describe religious phenomena in terms of neurobiological processes whose activity or inactivity they can observe with their brain scanners. Indeed, there might not be anything more to a religious experience than the activation of the right dorsal region of the hippocampus, or the inactivation of the top part of our parietal lobe (to name but two currently appealing hypotheses). On the other hand, perhaps these changes in brain activity that neuroscientists are observing with their modern scanners are simply the brain's response to an actual communication from God! After all, how else would your creator be able to communicate with you except by way of the sensory systems that your brain uses to experience reality?

MIXING HALLUCINOGENS

My students enjoy mixing their drugs in creative ways similar to what bartenders have done for alcoholic drinks. And to continue the parallel, they give their concoctions amusing names: "candy-flipping" is a combination of MDMA (ecstasy) followed by LSD; "hippy flipping" pairs two different psychedelic mushrooms; "kitty flipping" combines ketamine with MDMA, and "candy flipping on a string" is the trifecta combination of cocaine, LSD, and MDMA. I have no doubt that this list is not exhaustive. One of my students, a bright, intelligent, and devout young Muslim woman, admitted during class that she had been candy-flipping every weekend for the previous 2 years. She was convinced that the combination of these two hallucinogens was superior and more pleasant than either drug taken alone. I've heard this claim for many years and I find it hard to reconcile it with how scientists currently view the actions of hallucinogens in the brain. Why should taking a drug that kills serotonergic neurons—MDMA—actually enhance the actions of another drug—LSD—which requires the presence of serotonergic neurons? These anecdotal reports are fascinating and confirm my suspicion stated earlier: We do not currently understand how any hallucinogen works within our brain. This makes explaining this next phenomenon all the more difficult.

CHAPTER 6

Marijuana in the Brain

What drug is enjoyable and, under some circumstances, might actually be good for your brain? Can smoking this substance prevent age-related memory loss, for example? To answer these and similar questions, I turn now to a neurotransmitter system in the brain that was discovered through the use of one of the most common drugs in our history. This system may not have the most familiar of names—endogenous cannabinoid neurotransmitter—but the drug that tells us most about its function is certainly a household word: marijuana. Indeed, few drugs have the kind of colorful history that marijuana has achieved. Thus, before examining the neurotransmitter that it affects, let's look briefly at the story of the drug itself.

DOPE AND A ROPE

Among species of marijuana plants, *Cannabis indica* is the one grown principally for its psychoactive resins. It is likely a shorter, bushier version of the *Cannabis sativa*, which is used primarily for its fibers to make rope. Both plants, like catnip, contain active ingredients belonging to a family of compounds called terpenes, of which the primary psychoactive terpene is thought to be concentrated in the plants' resin as delta-9 tetrahydrocannabinol (THC). Initially investigated more than 100 years ago by two chemists, the Smith Brothers (William and Andrew) of later cough-drop fame, the plants contain approximately 50 cannabinoid-based compounds, with 4 major cannabinoids: trans-delta-9-THC and delta-8-THC, cannabidiol (the second most abundant psychoactive ingredient after THC), and cannabinol, which may be a decomposition product of THC that accumulates as cannabis samples age. After ingestion, the trans-delta-9-THC is converted in the liver to 11-hydroxy THC, which is equally potent and psychoactive.

Probably the oldest reference to the cannabis plant, in a pharmacy book from 2737 BCE, is related to its use as a medicine. The Chinese emperor Shen Nung (the Divine Farmer) referred to it as the "liberator of sin" and recommended it for the treatment of "female weakness," gout, rheumatism, malaria, constipation, and absent-mindedness. By 1000 BCE, its medicinal use, as indicated by available writings, had spread to India; by 500 BCE, it was familiar to the ancient Greeks.

The earliest reference to the use of cannabis as an inebriant was in 430 BCE, when the Greek historian Herodotus of Halicarnassus wrote that the Scythians burned the seeds and inhaled the smoke to induce intoxication during funerals. The plant is also mentioned several times (as "kaneh-bosem," קְנֵה-בֹשֶׂם) in the Old Testament (as Yahweh's instruction to Moses in Exodus 30:23) as a bartering material, incense, and an ingredient in holy anointing oil; it was likely used by the high priests of the temple as well as by Jesus. At that time in history, the word *messiah* simply meant "the anointed one." Use of the plant as an inebriant spread to the Muslim world and North Africa by 1000 CE and became epidemic by the 12th century. The exploring Spaniards likely brought kaneh-bos, by now probably pronounced as cannabis, to the New World in about 1545.

Meanwhile, let's not forget that other, more humdrum role that cannabis has played in history. English settlers brought it, as well as tobacco, to Jamestown, Virginia by 1611 and used its fibers to make rope. In the 1700s, George Washington grew cannabis on his farm and, according to entries in his diary, maintained a keen interest in cultivating better strains of the plant, evidently for the purpose of producing a better quality of rope. In 1942, the U.S. government made a number of movie-shorts aimed at encouraging farmers to plant hemp, or cannabis, for wartime use as rope. Other rather famous historical uses of cannabis fiber are said to include Chinese paper, the ropes and sails on Christopher Columbus's ships, the Declaration of Independence, World War II parachutes, and the first Levi jeans.

Today, when most people hear the term *marijuana*, they think of the leafy material from *C. indica* that is generally smoked. It contains 2% to 5% THC. Sinsemilla or ganja, made from the unpollinated female cannabis plant, may contain up to 15% THC. Hashish, which is actually the Arabic word for grass (which might explain the slang term for this plant), is made from a dried concentrate of the resin of cannabis flowers and contains about 8% to 14% THC. Hashish oil typically has from 15% to 60% THC, and bhang, a drink popular in India that is made of cannabis leaves, milk, sugar, and spices, has 2% to 5% THC. Kief (from the Arabic kaif كيف meaning "pleasure, well-being") is made from the dried resin of *C. indica* and usually has very high THC levels. Budder is a processed and concentrated form of hashish oil that is reported to contain between 82% and 99% THC by weight. Given its potency and effectiveness, it probably takes a lot of bread to buy this budder.

Whatever its form, marijuana is today categorized as a gateway drug for its role in leading users to try other illegal drugs. Overall, statistics show that very few young people use other illegal drugs without first trying marijuana. But the majority of marijuana users (about 60%) do not go on to use any other illicit drugs. By contrast, according to some statistics, most users report having tried legal substances—cigarettes or beer—before trying marijuana. Thus, tobacco and alcohol products could be considered gateway drugs as well. It's worth pointing out that that alcohol is considered as addictive as heroin, and tobacco is considered as addictive as crack cocaine.

What does marijuana do in the brain? It produces some excitatory behavioral changes, including euphoria, but it is not generally regarded as a stimulant. It can also produce some sedative effects, but not to the extent of a barbiturate or alcohol. It produces mild analgesic effects (pain relief) as well, but this action is not related pharmacologically to the pain-relieving effects of opiates or aspirin. Finally, marijuana produces hallucinations at high doses, but its structure does not resemble LSD or any other drug formally categorized as a hallucinogen. Thus, marijuana's effects on our body and brain are complex. Just how does it achieve these effects?

THE BRAIN'S OWN MARIJUANA-LIKE NEUROTRANSMITTER

The very high potency and structure of the cannabinoids contained within the marijuana plant enable them to cross the blood–brain barrier and bind to a receptor for the brain's very own endogenous cannabinoid neurotransmitter system. If this were not true, then the marijuana plant would be popular only for its use in making rope, paper, and cloth. The two currently identified neurotransmitter compounds (and there are probably more) in this system are anandamide, from the Sanskrit word *ananda* meaning "bliss," and 2-AG (2-arachidonoyl-glycerol). Unlike the other neurotransmitters that I've discussed, these two "endocannabinoids" are not stored in synaptic vesicles.

Rather, they are both produced within neurons and released to flow backward across the synapse to find their receptors, designated as CB1 and CB2. There are probably more of these CB receptors for marijuana in the human brain than for any other known neurotransmitter. The great abundance of these receptors and their widespread location gives an indication of the importance of the endocannabinoid system in the regulation of the brain's normal functioning.

Let's take a look at what these endocannabinoids do in the brain, to gain some insight into the consequences of smoking (or eating) marijuana. For example, anandamide inhibits the release of glutamate and acetylcholine within the cortex and hippocampus, an action that may underlie the ability of marijuana to impair one's capacity to form new memories when using the drug. The presence of cannabinoid receptors in the parts of the brain that control movement may explain the stumbling behavior that some marijuana users experience. Cannabinoid receptors greatly enhance the release of dopamine; this action plays a critical role in the ability of marijuana to produce euphoria. Finally, stimulation of cannabinoid receptors in the feeding centers of the hypothalamus may underlie the classic marijuana side effect known as the "munchies."

This last effect coincidentally drew the attention of scientists who conducted a series of clinical trials using a drug that blocks the brain's cannabinoid receptors. Their hope was that this drug's blocking action would produce an "anti-munchies" effect, thereby reducing food consumption and providing help to overweight patients. At first, the drug worked fairly well. People reported being less attracted to eating. Unfortunately, they also became severely depressed. What this discovery tells scientists is that our endogenous cannabinoid system is normally involved, either directly or indirectly, in elevating or controlling our mood and that antagonizing the cannabinoid receptors in the brain, as occurred with this novel drug, can produce some dangerous consequences.

In contrast, stimulating the brain's cannabinoid receptors may offer protection from the consequences of stroke, chronic pain, and neuroinflammation. Surprisingly, it may also protect against some aspects of age-associated memory loss. Ordinarily, we do not view marijuana as being good for our brain and certainly not for making memories. How could a drug that clearly impairs memory while people are under its sway protect their brains from the consequences of aging?

The answer likely has everything to do with the way that young and old brains function and the age-related changes in the actions of the neurotransmitters acetylcholine and glutamate. These two neurotransmitters are involved in making new memories and destroying old or unnecessary ones. Early in life, this process of creation and destruction is in balance, and so interfering with it—which occurs when using marijuana— might impair memory. But later in life, the roles of these neurotransmitters change in significant ways. In addition, the aged brain displays increasing evidence of inflammation and a dramatic decline in the production of new neurons, called neurogenesis. Marijuana may offer protection in at least three different ways: by preventing the damaging actions of glutamate, by reducing brain inflammation, and by restoring neurogenesis. Thus, later in life, marijuana might actually help your brain, rather than harm it. Research in my laboratory by Dr. Yannick Marchalant suggests that it takes very little marijuana to produce benefits in the older brain; his motto is "a puff is enough." The challenge for pharmacologists in the future will be to isolate the beneficial aspects of marijuana from its psychoactive effects, which themselves can be an additional burden to those suffering from the consequences of an aging brain.

Once again, the distribution of a neurotransmitter provides clues to its function in the brain. For example, our brains' endogenous cannabinoid neurons are in the hypothalamus feeding centers; when these receptors are stimulated, we feel hungry, and when they are blocked, we become less interested in eating. Cannabinoid neurons also influence the function of our cortex and various limbic (emotion-controlling) regions; when we stimulate these receptors, we impair higher cognitive functions as we experience euphoria, and when they are blocked, we feel depression. Because our brain appears to have a large number of different types of neurons that are affected by marijuana, a complete explanation of this drug's effects remains nearly impossible. What seems clear, however, is that the endogenous cannabinoid neurotransmitters that our brain produces do not appear to transmit information per se but appear to modulate how other neurotransmitter systems function. In this way, they act quite differently from the manner in which most other neu-rotransmitters behave.

MARIJUANA FOR MIGRAINES

Migraine sufferers have few options for reducing their headache pain, and most of the medications available have unpleasant side effects that limit their long-term usefulness. About 20 years ago a new class of drugs, the triptans, was introduced as an effective and safe alternative treatment. This class of drug works effectively for most patients but must be taken at the first sign of a headache. These drugs have their own unwanted side effects, such as feeling hot or cold, weak, or "strange" in some way. The strange feelings are often given the term *serotonin syndrome* and also include changes in mental status. These changes in mental status can be quite significant in individuals who carry a genetic vulnerability, such as people with bipolar illness or schizophre-nia. The assumption has been that these drugs work by acting upon serotonin receptors, which leads to a constriction of cere-bral blood vessels. This assumption may be incorrect.

One potentially important mechanism that was initially published in 1987 described how migraine headaches developed in some people shortly after they abruptly discontinued their long-term marijuana use. The implication was that marijuana was preventing the onset of migraines in vulnerable individuals. In addition, marijuana has long been known to possess analge-sic properties. Possibly, the marijuana was somehow masking the pain of the migraines. A recent publication from the

University of California, San Francisco, has offered a fascinating explanation for why the use of both triptans and marijuana prevents migraine headaches.

Our brain's own endogenous marijuana-like chemicals produce analgesia by modulating the entry of pain signals into the brain at the level of our spinal cord. Future generations of pain relievers will likely be developed on the basis of this action of marijuana in the body. The advantage of targeting the endogenous marijuana system is that only noxious or painful signals are blocked; normal touch sensation is normal.

This recent study made two significant advances: It confirmed the role of the endogenous marijuana neurotransmitter system as a potential target for treating migraines, and the results suggest that triptans may produce their migraine relief by activating the brain's own endogenous marijuana-like chemicals. This study may lead to the development of more effective migraine prevention and treatment. The challenge will be to find a dose of marijuana that produces pain relief without disturbing normal cognitive function.

MARIJUANA FOR THE TREATMENT OF PSYCHIC PAIN

The loss of someone you love hurts. Losing your job is painful. No one wants to be ignored because it brings on heartache and depression and possibly increases your chances of developing cancer or dementia. The field of psychoneuroimmunology has evolved to study the link between social and physical pain.

Obviously, to anyone who has experienced any of these events in life, the link between psychic and physical is quite real, and the symptoms are very difficult to treat.

During the evolution of our brain, those areas that were once only responsible for experiencing the sensory component of pain slowly evolved to provide the sensations associated with the emotional components of pain and its experience. We now respond with a psychic aching to social isolation that is often accompanied by a headache, nausea, depression, loss of appetite, and many other essential body functions. Recently, scientists speculated that because these two systems overlap functionally and anatomically in the brain, it might be possible to reduce social pain by targeting the physical pain experience with common over-the-counter drugs.

Two different types of common analgesics, acetaminophen and ibuprofen (i.e., Tylenol and Advil), are capable of producing this combined benefit by enhancing the action of the brain's endogenous marijuana neurotransmitters. A recent study demonstrated that regular marijuana use reduced the experience of low self-worth and the incidence of major depressive episodes in lonely people. This research supports the hypothesis that treating physical pain with simple over-the-counter drugs might lessen the psychic pain as well.

How are these simple over-the-counter drugs able to provide relief of psychic pain? They enhance the action of anandamide. Anandamide and the other marijuana-like chemicals in your brain are well known to control happiness and euphoria. Once anandamide is released inside your brain it is rather quickly inactivated by specific enzymes. One of these enzymes is called cyclooxygenase (COX). Ibuprofen and acetaminophen inhibit the function of COX. Thus, taking these drugs may enhance the actions of anandamide and thereby mimic the effects of marijuana in your brain. Obviously, their action in the brain must be rather subtle; otherwise these products would no longer be so easily available. Ultimately, targeting the biological mechanisms underlying the symptoms of loneliness might only require a trip to your corner drugstore.

CHAPTER 7

Simple Molecules That Turn You On and Off

W hy is a drug like PCP potentially lethal? Why does drinking alcohol make you drowsy? How do antianxiety drugs work, and why is it so dangerous to take them and alcohol at the same time? The answers to these questions have everything to do with the most abundant neurotransmitters in your brain, simple amino acids that are used for two simple functions: to turn on or turn off individual neurons. When used for communication, neurons usually respond to amino acid neurotransmitters—principally glutamate and GABA—with either excitation or inhibition. Glutamate is the principal excitatory amino acid neurotransmitter, whereas GABA is the principal inhibitory amino acid neurotransmitter.

GLUTAMATE: THE NEUROTRANSMITTER
THAT TURNS YOU ON

What is so important about glutamate? It makes and breaks connections between neurons, and it turns on other neurons to stimulate them into action. Glutamate neurotransmission is mediated through receptors that allow the passage of sodium or calcium ions into neurons; the receptors were named according to the chemical tools that were historically used to study them. For example, the subtype of glutamate receptors known as N-methyl-D-aspartate (NMDA) allows the entry of calcium ions into neurons. Following the entry of calcium ions, some truly interesting things begin to happen inside the neuron that leads to the production of what you might call a "memory." Calcium ions activate a complex cascade of biochemical changes that ultimately involve the genes of the neuron and that may actually change how the neuron behaves for the rest of your life. These biochemical changes may also alter how one neuron communicates with hundreds of other neurons.

Think of this neural process as a symphony of musicians playing together for the first time. Initially, everyone is playing his or her own song. Then the conductor arrives and hands out a musical score; all of the musicians begin to play in a complex pattern of rhythms that conveys information. Like the conductor, calcium ions entering via NMDA channels initiate the process of forming an ensemble of neuronal activity. Your neurons are the musicians, and when they become linked to each other according to some common pattern of activity, they form an ensemble that plays a particular song, or memory, which can recur only when that particular ensemble of neurons plays the same pattern together. In this analogy, memories can be seen as symphonies of activity in our brains, and just as we enjoy playing the same tunes over and over again, we also enjoy replaying pleasant memories. Unfortunately, glutamate's actions can prime us to play unpleasant or traumatic memories over and over again as well when they are triggered by innocent events in our daily lives.

In addition, the entry of calcium ions into neurons may sometimes become excessive as a result of aging, disease, or stroke and may initiate some harmful processes that may contribute to the removal of synapses or even the death of neurons. This information tells us quite a lot about the role of glutamate: When it works correctly, memories can be formed; when it does not work correctly, as when it induces too much calcium to enter the neuron, then death and destruction follow and memory is lost. Thus, maintaining a good balance of function related to the entry of calcium ions is a challenging but critical requirement for neurons, and the amino acid neurotransmitter glutamate plays a critical role in this process.

Glutamate also has a unique function in brain development. When you were very young, the neurons in your brain developed many connections, or synapses, with other neurons to optimize your ability to learn a great deal of information quickly, such as how to move your hands and feet, what your mother's voice sounds like, or what the color red looks like. But as you grew older (during adolescence), your brain became a bit like an overwired computer—for it to work better and faster, with less likelihood of failing, it became advantageous for it to remove unnecessary "wires," or connections. This is where glutamate's other unique abilities come into play. Your brain uses glutamate to prune synapses that have become unnecessary, which in turn allows the remaining neural circuits to function more efficiently. Later, when you're an adult, glutamate is critical for allowing your brain to be "plastic," to mold your responses to the environment so that you increase your chances of survival. Thus, like the Roman god Janus, the neurotransmitter glutamate has two faces: One is important for the early brain development and function in our past; the other is important for brain pruning and subsequent function in our future. Meanwhile, its staying power can sometimes be a mixed blessing. For example, as mentioned, traumatic memories formed through glutamate's actions can continue to haunt us long after the event that created those memories has occurred. The best example of this is called posttraumatic stress disorder; the unpleasant memories that characterize this disorder are very difficult to treat because of the amazing efficacy of glutamate to form lasting changes in the brain.

Currently, very few safe drugs are used clinically to target glutamate receptors. But there are two drugs of abuse, phencyclidine (aka PCP or angel dust) and ketamine, which can antagonize the NMDA type of glutamate receptor. Because these drugs block this principal excitatory neurotransmitter, they depress your brain's general level of activity. Your brain's information processing simply slows further and further until it can no longer keep you conscious. Phencyclidine was once used as an anesthetic, with some unfortunate consequences. Patients lost the ability to breathe, they became delirious and disoriented, and their heart rate decreased so much that they sometimes slipped into a coma and died.

Because phencyclidine is so potent, scientists believe that the brain makes its own endogenous PCP-like molecule, now named *angeldustin*, should it one day be isolated. Recent studies have suggested that reduced function of angeldustin may actually contribute to certain psychiatric syndromes, such as mania, and cause too much activity of the glutamate receptors in the brains of manic patients. Others have suggested that, whatever the cause, increased function of the brain's principal excitatory neurotransmitter drives the symptoms of mania such as racing thoughts, insomnia, and impulsiveness. That said, the medical treatment of mania, usually with the use of a salt called lithium chloride, does not involve reducing neuronal functioning of glutamate but instead slows the manic brain by very different mechanisms. One of these mechanisms may be related to lithium's ability to induce the birth of new GABA-releasing neurons, of which the brains of manic patients have a reduced number. This possibility would make sense given the particular nature of that neurotransmitter. In any case, too much inhibition of glutamate would severely impair the brain's ability to process information. Our brains need to have glutamate's excitatory actions working appropriately for us to learn and pay attention. Rather than reduce an overactive brain by using drugs that inhibit glutamate, humans have discovered many different drugs that force our brains to slow down by stimulating the function of GABA neurons.

GAMMA-AMINOBUTYRIC ACID (GABA): THE NEUROTRANSMITTER THAT TURNS YOU OFF

In contrast to glutamate, the amino acid neurotransmitter GABA turns neurons off. After being released into the synaptic space, it binds to a protein receptor. The best studied of these is the GABAA receptor, and drugs that bind to it enhance the ability of GABA to stabilize the activity of the neuron. In so doing, these drugs have produced dramatic therapeutic benefits for a wide range of disorders, particularly for the treatment of anxiety and insomnia. Why should this be the case? There are two simple reasons: GABA receptors are widely distributed throughout all brain regions, and GABA is virtually always inhibitory. So any drug that enhances GABA receptor function produces an overall decrease in the activity of neurons everywhere in your brain. Contrary to the claims made in popular magazines, you cannot accomplish this effect simply by eating GABA-containing substances to increase the amount of GABA in your brain. While floating in the bloodstream, ingested GABA becomes electrically charged, preventing it from passing across the blood–brain barrier. Taking a few hundred milligrams of GABA every day, therefore, will not reduce your anxiety or help you sleep. Instead, your treatments of choice should be drugs that turn on your existing GABA receptors so they can turn off your brain—either a little to reduce your anxiety or a lot to make you sleep.

Although recent evidence suggests that anxiety, like depression and migraine headaches, may be related to the dysfunction of serotonin receptors more than to GABA, medical science prefers to treat anxiety with prescription, GABA-enhancing drugs, which do work to reduce this symptom. What do the actions of these drugs tell us about the causes of anxiety in the brain? Not that much. Again, simply because it is possible to treat the symptoms of a disorder by manipulating a particular neurotransmitter system in the brain does not tell us anything about the actual cause of the disorder. All we can say with certainty is that if you're feeling anxious, taking one of these drugs will make you feel less so.

ENHANCING THE ACATION OF GABA WITH FOOD AND DRUGS

Among the earliest antianxiety treatments were drugs that simply made you sleepy—these drugs essentially depress activity in the brain and make it difficult to feel anything at all. Various salts made from the common element bromine were used to reduce brain activity associated with epilepsy, anxiety, or stress. Fans of old movies set in a bygone era may remember the occasional actress holding her forehead and stating that she needed to "take a Bromo" to treat a headache. Although these salts were effective at reducing the neural activity in the brain that is required to experience pain, or to even maintain wakefulness, they were extremely toxic to the kidneys and ultimately removed from the commercial market. They were replaced by opiates, which were available without restriction during the 18th and 19th centuries. So was a more popular and socially acceptable drug that in many cultures, including our own, still has almost iconic status today.

ALCOHOL

Alcohol (ethyl, not methyl) may have been the first anxiety-reducing agent. There is evidence that distillation of grains to make alcohol-containing beverages, what today we would refer to as beer, may have begun in the Fertile Cresent (between present-day Iran, Iraq, Syria, and Israel) by about 10,000 BCE. The ancient Egyptians also produced alcoholic beverages, referring in some passages within their texts to the social problems associated with drunkenness. Other Egyptian texts, written around 1600 BCE, contained 100 different medical prescriptions calling for the use of alcohol. Over subsequent centuries, several types of alcohol, distilled and fermented, were developed, and they all had their calming effects.

Alcohol has two principal actions in the brain. First, it enhances the widespread inhibitory effects of the neurotransmitter GABA and acts as a depressant on the entire central nervous system. For this reason, in the 19th century, alcohol was widely used as a general anesthetic. Unfortunately, the duration of its depressant action on the brain was too long and could not be controlled easily or safely. The effective dose for surgical analgesia using alcohol is very close to its lethal dose. Therefore, it was possible to induce sufficient anesthesia in a cowboy for a surgeon to remove an arrow from a leg, but it was unlikely that the unfortunate cowboy would survive the operation. Thus, if the arrow didn't kill him, the operation certainly might. Of course, prior to the 20th century, this was generally true of most medicines. Now you understand why Hippocrates requested in his oath that physicians, at the very least, do no harm. Drug therapies in ancient times often produced more harm than benefit to the patient.

In addition to its actions on GABA receptors, alcohol inhibits the brain's principal excitatory neurotransmitter system, glutamate. Given glutamate's critical role in making memories, this inhibitory effect may underlie the amnesia that is often associated with intoxication—that is, the classic blackout. It may also explain the inappropriate behavior that often occurs when people drink. The consumption of only modest amounts of alcohol produces an apparent stimulation of the brain that may result in unrestrained activity of various brain regions caused by the lessening of their inhibitory controls. Which behaviors are released from control first? Usually, alcohol consumption initially releases what are called "punished behaviors," such as not drinking and driving, not dancing on picnic tables naked in the park at midnight, etc. You get the idea: These are behaviors that we are warned against undertaking by your mom, the police, or God.

As with most drugs that affect your brain, the rate at which your blood alcohol levels rise also affect your behavior—that is, faster changes in blood alcohol levels produce more dramatic effects on your behavior. As alcohol levels increase, more and more of your brain is turned off by alcohol's enhancement of GABA. Ultimately, when blood levels become too high, neurons critical to controlling your breathing and heart rate are inactivated because of overstimulation of their GABA receptors. Therefore, death resulting from alcohol intoxication occurs because you stop breathing. Usually, before that happens, your brain's vomiting control center will become activated at blood alcohol levels of about 0.12%. However, if you drink slowly and steadily, you can sneak up on these protective neurons and inactivate them with alcohol. Once this happens, your body makes no effort to rid itself of alcohol in the stomach by vomiting and the levels of alcohol in your blood can continue to rise to lethal levels. Thus, vomiting at the end of the party is a good thing, really. Your body is trying to protect you.

There is ample evidence that alcohol was tested in ancient times for its potential benefits beyond being a source of nutrition. Unfortunately, the side effects usually greatly outweighed the benefits. Alcohol alters the activity of neurons that project into the cerebellum, a structure that is critical for the timing and execution of smooth movements. This leads to the incoordination that is seen in people after drinking alcoholic beverages.

Finally, our drinking behavior is greatly influenced by our environment. The people who make a profit on the sale of alcoholic beverages are well aware of this fact and clearly take advantage of the knowledge in designing their environments. When studies were made of the behavior of people in bars, time was a big predictor of alcohol abuse; for example, the shorter the stay in the bar the faster the rate of consumption. People drinking alone stayed the shortest time and drank the most; thus there are always plenty of single (usually uncomfortable) barstools available. One study compared drinking behavior in two different settings, a rock & roll bar and a country & western bar. The study found a correlation between the sipping rate and the beats per minute of the music. Fast-paced music was associated with the slowest drinking rate. Music that was closest to a person's resting heart rate produced the fastest drinking. Lyrics of slow songs also contributed to drinking behavior. Tear-jerk lonesome country & western lyrics involving losing, hurting, and cheating, or working, dying, and drinking, or wailing and self-pitying were associated with increased drinking—who's not surprised?! Live bands and action photography flashing on the walls also increased drinking rates. Next time you find yourself in such an environment, take notice of how carefully and subtly your behavior is being controlled so that you'll spend the most amount of money in the shortest period of time.

BARBITURATES

At the end of the 19th century, it was obvious that an alternative drug for anxiety was necessary that would be safer than the popular and highly available alcohol and opium. In 1904, the first barbiturate, barbital, was introduced and sold as Veronal. It was a nontoxic sedative, and because of its anticonvulsant properties, it also appeared to be ideal for treating and preventing the symptoms of epilepsy. As you might have guessed already, barbiturates reduce neural activity in the brain by enhancing the function of GABA receptors and producing widespread synaptic inhibition, just like alcohol.

Just how safe the barbiturates are is subject to much debate. For one thing, in high doses, they are lethal, the reason that for many years barbiturate overdose was a common way by which people committed suicide. In addition, the rebound produced by withdrawal from barbiturates is characterized by increased neural activity throughout the brain, leading to symptoms that are often the motivation for taking these drugs in the first place, such as anxiety, disorientation, hallucinations, convulsions, insomnia, tachycardia, or nightmares. The fact that alcohol can prevent the withdrawal symptoms of barbiturates shows the commonality of their action at the GABA receptor. This commonality underlies the reason that alcohol and barbiturates produce a synergistic toxicity in the brain. What this means is that these drugs should never be taken together because their effects will be compounded, or even multiplied, and can induce a dramatic and possibly permanent loss of higher brain function, leading to a vegetative state or coma. This array of potentially life-threatening risks associated with barbiturates led to the introduction of an entirely new class of antianxiety medications to the market.

BENZODIAZEPINES

The first benzodiazepine, chlordiazepoxide, was initially synthesized in 1947 and first sold commercially in 1960 as Librium (because it produced an emotional equilibrium). Shortly thereafter, diazepam was sold as Valium (Latin for "be strong and well") and quickly became the most prescribed antianxiety drug in the Western world. Both of these drugs are converted into other psychoactive agents within the brain and body. Some of these metabolites were isolated from the urine of people taking Valium and Librium and were discovered to be quite effective new drugs that could reduce anxiety and produce sleepiness. Because of changes in fat solubility, these newer drugs acted on the brain faster and, as typically follows, had a shorter duration of action. They are generally safe to use in controlled doses, but once again, withdrawal from them produces abrupt increases in widespread neural activity that is often expressed as insomnia and anxiety. Recently, an even newer class of drugs called non-benzodiazepines was introduced to consumers, and these drugs also reduce anxiety and induce sleepiness.

All of these drugs, benzodiazepine and non-benzodiazepine alike, exert their effects only in the presence of GABA, enhancing the action of GABA at its receptor. The highest concentration of these receptors is found in the neocortex, hippocampus, cerebellum, and throughout the limbic system (which is involved in producing both pleasant and unpleasant emotional responses). The presence of these receptors within the hippocampus may explain why benzodiazepines can produce amnesia. They may inactivate the neural circuits in this structure that are critical for the consolidation of memories.

Recent studies suggest that the brain may contain its own family of valium-like compounds, the beta-carbolines. Some of these antagonize GABA function and others enhance it, but all may share a similar ability to inhibit the destruction of the neurotransmitters dopamine, norepinephrine, and serotonin; taken together, these effects would tend to produce a mild, relaxed euphoria. The balance of action of these endogenous antianxiety compounds is determined by the genes we inherit from our parents, which control the carbolines produced and probably predispose us to being anxious or laidback throughout our lives. It is now thought that anxiety disorders may be related to a dysfunction of GABA receptors and the balance of function of these carbolines.

Indeed, scientists have speculated that the brains of people who suffer from generalized anxiety disorder may produce too many of these chemicals from their diet. True, some carbolines can be formed spontaneously from the constituents of our diet. For example, coffee produces beta-carbolines, and alcohol can be converted by bacterium in the gut, *Helicobacter pylori*, to form a beta-carboline. Whether these exogenous beta-carbolines are produced in sufficient quantities to produce functional consequences in the brain remains to be determined. We do know, however, that the carbolines in the brain are similar to those found, for example, in the *Banisteriopsis caapi* vine; extracts of the vine are a key ingredient in the mildly psychoactive sacramental beverage Ayahuasca from the Amazon. Because the ingredients in these vines, known as harmala alkaloids, resemble molecules used by your brain, their consumption can influence how you think and feel. It perhaps stands to reason then, if not yet confirmed in fact, that consuming exogenous beta-carbolines to correct an endogenous imbalance of these molecules would have a similar influence on the brain.

INHIBITING THE ACTION OF GABA

What would it feel like if you ingested a drug that blocked the brain's most important inhibitory neurotransmitter? Would you become excited? Thujone is such a drug; it blocks the action of GABA at one of its principal receptors in the brain. Thujone can be found in many different plants, but it is most often associated with wormwood (*Artemisia absinthium*), the extract of which, when mixed with alcohol, produces a bright green drink called absinthe. During the mid-1800s, this drink became very popular in Europe, especially among such artists as Manet, Degas, Toulouse-Lautrec, and Van Gogh. The ritual was to pour the emerald-green liquid slowly over sugar held in a perforated spoon and then dilute it with water. The taste was very bitter, and the drink was said to produce a "lucid drunkenness." Then, during the late 1800s, studies by the French psychiatrist Valentin Magnan discovered that wormwood oil produced inappropriately increased brain activity—in short, an epileptic reaction. Thus, it was thought that the effects of chronic use of absinthe, such as contractions of the face muscles and extremities, anxiety, paranoia, energy loss, numbness, headaches, delirium, paralysis, and death, resulted from the existence of thujone in the wormwood extract used in this drink. One author in the *American Journal of Pharmacy* wrote in 1868 that "it's an ignoble poison, destroying life not until it has more or less brutalized its votaries, and made driveling idiots of them." A campaign against thujone ensued and resulted, by the early 20th century, in the banning of absinthe in many countries, including in the United States.

Today, however, it is known that the manner in which absinthe was once prepared would have produced only very low levels of thujone in a typical serving. Therefore, the symptoms noted among chronic users of absinthe more likely resulted from the excessive consumption of improperly distilled spirits rather than from the effects of thujone. To be sure, thujone is a GABA antagonist and can produce excitatory effects in small doses, but these effects are mild. It can be found in very low amounts in drinks such as vermouth (from the German *Wermuth* for wormwood), chartreuse, and Bénédictine. Of course, it remains in similarly small amounts in absinthe, the legal sale of which has now resumed in most countries.

CHAPTER 8

Remnants of an Ancient Past

Very primitive multicellular organisms, such as the hydra (e.g., *Chlorohydra viridissima*, the ultimate simple feeding tube), have nervous systems that may only use simple proteins as neurotransmitters, suggesting that these proteins were the first signaling molecules used by primordial nervous systems. If we extract a few of these proteins from the "brain" of a typical hydra and inject them in human neurons, they will actually produce similar signaling responses from those neurons.

In fact, the proteins used by hydra in their nervous systems are identical to some of the proteins that our brains use to help us think and feel. These proteins are called neuropeptides. A neuropeptide is like a string of beads, and each bead is an amino acid. Neuropeptides may be assembled from only a few or from hundreds of different amino acids. Your body contains many different types of neuropeptides that are assembled from the amino acids found in your diet. Neurons that produce and release these neuropeptides are found throughout the body and brain and influence a diverse array of body functions, including the release of hormones and the absorption of nutrients from our blood.

The evolutionary history of our neuropeptides is quite interesting and tells us a great deal about their current role and why they are found in certain places in the body and not others. One very important neuropeptide is insulin, which is produced by the pancreas. Some neuroscientists have speculated that an insulin-like peptide might have been the principal ancestor to many of our other neuropeptides that are still structurally related to each other. For example, growth hormone and prolactin, peptides that control breast development and milk production, respectively, may have diverged from a common ancestor about 350 million years ago. Therefore, it's not surprising that growth and nursing are also closely related to each other. As studies of mammals and hydra have demonstrated, evolution does not tinker with some molecules. If something works well, it tends to stay around and continue to be used across eons of time.

Alternatively, some neuropeptides have been modified only slightly but often for related purposes. For example, most animal venoms are derived from neuropeptide-related precursors, and some may have originated from brain peptides that initially appeared at least 100 million years ago and have since been undergoing modification and mutation. Yet, some venoms still retain the ability to perform functions that their evolutionary parent molecule still performs, such as an insulin-like ability to control blood glucose levels. Because of this shared evolutionary history, venoms extracted from species that range from very simple single-celled organisms to very complex animals and plants have become popular tools for scientists studying how human neuropeptide neurons function. During the past 30 years, these studies have demonstrated that there are more than 100 different neuropeptide neurotransmitters in our brain and body. These neuropeptides are found at very low concentrations and are very potent.

This chapter focuses on neuropeptide neurotransmitters whose actions in the brain were discovered through the euphoric and pain-relieving effects of one of the most powerful and addicting class of drugs ever known. By way of contrast, it also discusses the pain-relieving effects of a few drugs that do not work through these neuropeptides but, rather, through a very different mechanism. The contrast is interesting in what it tells us about these neuropeptides in the context of the full arsenal of mechanisms that the body uses to protect itself from pain and other distress.

OPIATES AND OPIATE-LIKE NEUROTRANSMITTERS

The euphoric and sleep-producing effects of opiates, which are derived from the poppy plant, were well known to ancient civilizations. Around 4000 BCE, for example, the Sumerians (Babylonians) carved pictures of the poppy plant into tablets inscribed with the words *hul* ("joy") and *gil* ("plant"). In the classical literature of Virgil (first century BCE), Somnus, the Roman god of sleep (a translation of the Greek Hypnos), was sometimes described as carrying poppies and an opium container from which he poured juice into the eyes of the sleeper. Chinese legend has the poppy plant springing up from the earth where the Buddha's eyelids had fallen after he cut them off to prevent sleep.

The first specific medical use of opium was described in the Ebers papyrus of ancient Egypt (about 1500 BCE), where it is presented as a remedy for excessive crying in children. The substance was important for Greek medicine as well. According to Galen, the last of the great Greek physicians (second century CE), opium was an antidote to poison and venoms and cured headaches, vertigo, deafness, blindness, muteness, coughs, colic, and jaundice. He also noted its recreational use at the time, commenting on the widespread sale of opium cakes and candies.

Various opium preparations, usually as extractions into some type of alcoholic beverage, were later developed, including Dr. Thomas Sydenham's version of laudanum during the 17th century, which contained 2 ounces of strained opium, 1 ounce of saffron, and a dram of cinnamon and cloves dissolved in a pint of Canary wine. The 19th century author Thomas De Quincey purchased laudanum for a toothache and then spent the rest of his life taking the drug and writing about his experiences with it (*Confessions of an English Opium-Eater*, 1821). Another preparation was paregoric, a combination of opium, camphor, and anise oil that was developed in the mid-20th century for the treatment of diarrhea in infants.

Meanwhile, in about 1806, when working as a pharmacist's apprentice in Paderborn, Germany, Friedrich Sertürner isolated the primary active ingredient in opium and named it morphium, after Morphius, the Greek god of dreams and the son of Hypnos. Later investigations discovered an additional active ingredient called codeine, the Greek word for "poppy head." In 1874, chemists attached two acetyl groups to morphine and produced heroin, which Bayer Labs marketed in 1898 as a supposedly nonaddicting substitute for codeine. The two additional acetyl groups made heroin more potent than morphine because they increased its fat solubility and allowed more of the drug to enter the brain very rapidly. Heroin is, in short, just a chemical trick to get morphine into the brain faster. But once inside the brain, heroin can do nothing on its own. First, it must be converted into morphine by enzymes that remove those two additional acetyl groups. Then, as the molecule originally found in the poppy seed, it can act to produce pain relief or euphoria.

The effects of morphine, codeine, and heroin in the brain are dose related. Small doses produce drowsiness, decreased anxiety and inhibition, reduced concentration, muscle relaxation, pain relief, depressed respiration, constricted pupils, nausea, and a decreased cough reflex, which is why codeine found its way into cough suppressants. At slightly higher doses, morphine and heroin can produce a state of intense elation or euphoria. Their euphorigenic property is related to their speed of entry into the brain, which again is directly related to their fat solubility. The euphoric effect is most enhanced by injecting these drugs into a vein, thus greatly accelerating their entry into the brain, and results in the "kick, bang, or rush" that addicts describe as an abdominal orgasm, a sudden flush of warmth localized in the pit of the stomach. Interestingly, the user does not experience this rush if the drug is smoked, sniffed, or swallowed, because of the much slower absorption and entry into the brain via these methods of administration.

As always, the Law of Initial Value determines how a person responds to a drug. For example, in well-adjusted, emotionally stable, pain-free people, morphine may produce restlessness and anxiety. In contrast, elation most often occurs in users who are either abnormally depressed or highly excited. At very high doses of morphine, the profound depression of brain activity deepens into a state of unconsciousness that can be fatal. Respiratory depression caused by inhibition of the brain's breathing centers is the ultimate cause of death.

The effects of morphine eventually led many scientists to predict that the brain possesses its own endogenous opiate-like neurotransmitters and its own complement of endogenous opiate receptors in the brain. In the mid-1970s research confirmed that the brain and body do indeed contain some endogenous morphine-like peptides and christened them "endorphins." These peptides control our experience of pain by stopping the flow of pain signals into our brains, and this action is enhanced by the taking of opiate drugs like morphine, as well as by engaging in activities (e.g., jogging) that can produce an "endorphin high."

Our ancestors were intimately aware of the beneficial effects of other plant extracts for the treatment of pain. For example, myrrh—isolated from the dried resin in the bark of *Commiphora myrrha*, a shrub found in Somalia and throughout the Middle East—was historically used in liniments, including in Chinese medicine, to treat the symptoms of arthritis and as an antiseptic ointment. It may be slightly more potent than morphine and may act via central endogenous opiate receptors to produce pain relief. Another resin, frankincense, can be extracted from the *Boswellia sacra* tree and exhibits a mild anti-inflammatory action similar to that of aspirin. In ancient times, frankincense and myrrh were commonly used together as a salve to relieve postpartum pain and to reduce bleeding after delivery. They were also burned as incense and, as immortalized in the Christmas story of the three wise men, were highly valued as a gift.

Our ancestors were, of course, ignorant of the neurobiology of opiates or how pain was produced in the human body. In the distant past, when a person felt pain—particularly in the absence of evidence of injury—spiritual healers or medicine men developed fanciful myths to explain the cause of the pain, treated it with a decoction from the willow tree or myrrh shrub, and were often rewarded with elevated positions in their communities when their treatments seemed to magically make the pain go away and produced such an intense feeling of joy at the same time. With the advent of modern science, we know more about the mechanisms of pain and about the reasons why some drugs are better at treating pain than others.

Morphine-like proteins, as well as many other psychoactive chemicals capable of acting on the brain's neurotransmitter receptors, may also originate from many commonly consumed foods, including milk; eggs; cheese; grains such as rice, wheat, rye, and barley; spinach; mushrooms; pumpkin; meat; and various fish such as tuna, sardine, herring, and salmon. Dairy products in particular contain a protein known as casein, which enzymes in your intestines can easily convert into beta-caseomorphine. When newborns start nursing, the beta-caseomorphine can easily pass out of the immature gut and into the brain (both are still lacking viable barriers at this young age) and produce euphoria. The pleasurable feeling produced by this heroin-like compound in newborn mammals after their first taste of mother's milk is believed to encourage the infant to return again and again for nourishment. Adults do not experience this euphoria after drinking milk because of the intact blood–gut and blood–brain barriers. Perhaps if we could experience the euphoria of heroin and the pain relief of morphine with each glass of milk, then dairy cows would only be sold on the black market! Finally, because so many of my students ask this question every year: The opiate-containing poppy seeds consumed as part of a morning muffin or bagel have no pain-relieving or other psychoactive effect because the dose is far too low. Nonetheless, it is possible to detect traces of morphine and codeine in the urine within a few hours after consumption. Keep that in mind during your next job interview process.

The universally feared gluten grains (wheat, barley, and rye) produce a related compound in the gut, called gluteomorphin. In addition, these grains are capable of damaging the lining of the intestinal tract and lead to the malabsorption of calcium, iron, B complex vitamins and vitamin C, and trace minerals, including zinc, magnesium, and boron. This impaired absorption, also called the leaky gut syndrome, may contribute greatly to the ill health of the brain (and immune system); however, whether these changes lead to cognitive changes induced specifically by gluteomorphin is currently unknown.

CHAPTER 9

_____

SLEEPING VERSUS WAKING

W hy do treatments for the symptoms of the common cold make us drowsy? How does coffee work? This chapter touches briefly on neurotransmitters whose actions in the brain affect our sleep–wake cycle and on a few well-known substances that block these effects. One such neurotransmitter is histamine, whose neurons influence our level of arousal throughout the day. Over-the-counter antihistamine medications used to treat allergies and cold symptoms block histamine receptors and interfere with the ability of this neurotransmitter to keep one aroused and awake. The result is drowsiness. Meanwhile, because GABA neurons induce sleepiness by turning off histamine and acetylcholine neurons, any drug that enhances the action of GABA (e.g., alcohol, barbiturates, or Valium) is going to be synergistic with the over-the-counter antihistamine drugs. Thus, if taken together, these two kinds of drugs can bring about a life-threatening depression in brain activity.

ADENOSINE

This neurotransmitter has diverse functions throughout the brain that are also related to our sleep–wake cycles. We know a lot about it because of the ready availability of a very safe, highly effective adenosine receptor antagonist that is served hot or cold, with or without cream, throughout the world—caffein-ated coffee. Caffeine is also commonly found with theophylline (a molecule that is very similar to caffeine) in tea. Indeed, although caffeine is found in at least 63 plant species, 54% of the world's consumption derives from just two different beans, *Coffea arabica* and *Coffea robusta*, and 43% derives from the tea plant *Camellia sinensis*.

Coffee is rich in biologically active substances such as trigo-nelline, quinolinic acid, tannic acid, and pyrogallic acid. The vitamin niacin is formed in great amounts from trigonelline during the coffee bean roasting process. Coffee is also a rich source of antioxidants. Various ingredients in coffee beans con-tribute to aspects of the drink—for example, its bitterness— that people find either appealing or unpleasant. Recently, some entrepreneurs have found a way to remove the bitterness by "fil-tering" coffee beans through the gastrointestinal tract of the Asian palm civet, *Paradoxurus hermaphroditus*. The civets, nocturnal omnivores that are about the size of a cat, eat the beans, which then pass through the animals' gastrointestinal systems undigested but presumably not unaffected. The beans are then extracted from the animals' stool, cleaned up, and sold. It's hardly an enticing process, but the claim is that the animal's digestive enzymes metabolize the proteins that cause the bitter taste of the coffee bean. Although this is certainly possible, the novel flavor of the beans is just as likely a result of the bean's absorption of some of the less appealing contents of the animals' gut.

Coffee drinking (or consuming caffeine from non-coffee sources) has been associated with a significantly lowered risk of developing Parkinson's disease. The neuroprotective effect requires about five to six cups of coffee per day for many years and appears to be mostly beneficial only to males. Women benefit from coffee-drinking in other ways, particularly with regard to a reduced incidence of type 2 diabetes.

Nonfiltered, boiled coffee, in contrast to filtered coffee, actually increases serum levels of the bad cholesterol LDL without affecting blood levels of the good cholesterol HDL. Thus, it appears that the constituents of coffee may alter the way we metabolize and distribute our fat. Does this translate into a removal of fat from around the waist? A group of scientists at the University of Southern Queensland in Toowoomba, Australia, attempted to answer this question. When obese diabetic rats were given caffeine for 30 weeks, their ability to regulate blood sugar and insulin levels improved; unfortunately, the level of cholesterol in their blood increased significantly. Rats placed on cafeteria-style diets high in carbohydrates and fat developed symptoms of the now infamous metabolic syndrome, characterized by obesity, hypertension, impaired glucose tolerance, cardiovascular damage, and fatty liver and elevated blood lipids. Daily coffee intake (equal to about five cups of regular brewed coffee per day) significantly benefited these rats by improving the health of their cardiovascular system, lowering blood pressure, and improving liver function and glucose tolerance. The contractility of their heart muscle improved in a way that resembled the hypertrophy often seen in athletes where the heart actually becomes more efficient.

Overall, people who drink substantial amounts of coffee daily tend to live longer than people who do not. In addition, recent evidence suggests that moderate coffee-drinking of about two to three cups each day might reduce your chance of developing Alzheimer's disease. What is the connection between coffee, diabetes, and diseases of the brain? No one is sure, but elevated insulin levels in the blood may be a critical link, because type 2 diabetes makes both men and women more likely to develop both Parkinson's and Alzheimer's disease.

Many people drink coffee to reduce drowsiness. How does caffeine achieve this effect in the brain? The answer begins with a consideration of the function of the acetylcholine neurons that control your ability to pay attention. Adenosine negatively controls the activity of these neurons, meaning that when adenosine binds to its receptor on acetylcholine neurons, their activity slows. The production and release of adenosine in your brain is linked to metabolic activity while you are awake. Therefore, the concentration of adenosine in the neighborhood of acetylcholine neurons increases constantly while your brain is active during the day. As the levels of adenosine increase, they steadily inhibit your acetylcholine neurons, your brain's activity gradually slows, and you begin to feel drowsy and ultimately fall asleep. Caffeine comes to the rescue because it, like theophylline from tea, is a potent blocker of adenosine receptors and, therefore, of the adenosine-driven drowsiness and sleep. One can take this too far, however. One of my students decided to test these caffeine effects by ingesting a packet of instant coffee, right out of the box. He reported that he enjoyed eating it so much that he decided to finish off the entire container of 32 packets! Three days later, he stopped having explosive diarrhea and finally fell asleep completely exhausted.

Given everything that you've read about drugs that produce a rewarding and euphoric feeling, you might suspect that coffee also somehow affects dopamine neurons. You would be correct. Caffeine sets free the activity of dopamine neurons to bring euphoria and bliss to every cup of coffee or every glass of cola. Most cans of cola contain about 40 milligrams of caffeine; therefore, most teenagers consume as much caffeine as their parents—the only thing that differs is the vehicle for the drug. The widespread availability of foods containing caffeine has led experts to suggest that 80% of all people in North America have measureable levels of caffeine in their brains from embryo to death.

WHY DOES COFFEE MAKE US FEEL SO GOOD?

We all remember that first cup of coffee; it tasted terrible. It was too hot, too bitter, and maybe too sweet, but it offered the promise of alertness after a night of poor sleep. The wonderful thing about coffee is that it delivered on its promise every time; subsequently, you've never been able to walk away from it. If you've ever faced giving up on caffeinated coffee to lessen the symptoms of fibrocystic breast disease or the tremors associated with Parkinson's disease, you know well the craving that can develop. Why does this happen? Two reasons: Scientists have known for many years that coffee stimulates the release of the neurotransmitter dopamine. Dopamine produces the euphoria and pleasant feelings that people often associate with their first cup of coffee in the morning. Many drugs that produce euphoria, such as cocaine, amphetamine, and ecstasy, act upon dopamine in the brain. This action by coffee has always been an adequate explanation for why caffeine is the most widely consumed psychoactive substance in the world.

But do we all really just crave more arousal? Is being more aroused enough to explain why for some people coffee is akin to cocaine—they crave it constantly and will work hard to have a supply always at hand? One of my students claimed that he regularly consumed two full pots of coffee (equivalent to about 20 cups of coffee!) every morning before coming to class. He indicated that he knew it was time to stop when the tremors in his hands became impossible to control.

This student's experience reminds me of the verses of the French novelist Honoré de Balzac: "This coffee plunges into the stomach…the mind is aroused, and ideas pour forth like the battalions of the Grand Army on the field of battle.…Memories charge at full gallop…the light cavalry of comparisons deploys itself magnificently; the artillery of logic hurry in with their train of ammunition; flashes of wit pop up like sharp-shooters." To me, these behaviors suggest a level of addiction that goes beyond the simple enhancement of one neurotransmitter system.

A recent report by a group of scientists from Rome outlined how coffee's addictive properties also involve the brain's marijuana-like neurotransmitter system. This is how it all seems to work. When you first started drinking coffee, the arousal was all you wanted and also all that you got. Still, being more attentive and vigilant was all you needed to get through the day. As you continued drinking coffee, your liver compensated for the additional chemicals in your diet by becoming more efficient at metabolizing the caffeine. Your brain also made some adjustments. Ultimately, you needed more and more coffee each day to achieve the same level of arousal and vigilance. While all of this was occurring, something else far more mysterious was happening inside your brain: Caffeine had begun stimulating your brain's endogenous marijuana neurotransmitter system. These biochemical adjustments introduced an entirely new level of pleasure to your morning cup of java. In addition, it made avoiding that third or fourth cup of coffee even harder to accomplish. But there is a surprise ending to this tale.

DECAF COFFEE IS JUST AS GOOD FOR YOU

It's the end of the day and you've failed to consume the recommended amount of coffee to prevent Parkinson's and Alzheimer's disease or prostate cancer or diabetes. Maybe it's time to settle down with a cup of decaffeinated coffee. However, does decaffeinated coffee offer the same health benefits as caffeinated coffee? The answer is a qualified yes. Fortunately, with or without the caffeine, coffee is rich in biologically active substances such as phenols that exhibit both antioxidant and anticarcinogenic properties. Some studies suggest that certain oils produced when coffee beans are roasted may favorably affect blood-sugar control by enhancing the action of insulin to remove sugar from the blood. Trigonelline—molecule of niacin with a methyl group attached—may help to prevent dental caries by preventing the bacteria *Streptococcus mutans* from adhering to teeth. Trigonelline is unstable above 160 degrees F; the methyl group detaches, unleashing the niacin (vitamin B3). The vitamin niacin is formed in great amounts from trigonelline during the coffee bean roasting process. Two or three espressos can provide half your recommended daily allowance and may be responsible for lowering blood cholesterol.

Chlorogenic acid is an antioxidant whose actions may underlie the presumed ability of coffee to prevent type 2 diabetes mellitus. It can reduce the production of glucose by the liver and also lessen the hyperglycemic peak in the blood following the consumption of sugar. The plant is believed to use this chemical to defend itself from viruses, bacteria, and fungi; it may provide the same benefits for humans.

Ferulic acid is an antioxidant that neutralizes free radicals and may prevent oxidative damage to our bodies caused by exposure to ultraviolet light when we unwisely do not use sunscreens. Ferulic acid can also decrease blood glucose levels and reduce the level of cholesterol and triglyceride; these actions may underlie the potential benefits of coffee drinking, decaffeinated or not. Caffeinated coffee has been shown to increase blood pressure and may pose a health threat to people with cardiovascular disease; fortunately, decaffeinated coffee does not pose this risk.

COFFEE OR TEA: WHICH IS BETTER?

The cognitive decline of a large group of people who regularly consume coffee or tea (about five cups of each beverage per week) was monitored for 9 years. Overall, the tea drinkers exhibited a slower rate of cognitive decline than the coffee drinkers but the difference was rather modest. Therefore, the best advice may have been offered by the 19th-century Dutch physician Buntckuh, who advised "men and women to drink tea daily, hour by hour if possible; beginning with ten cups a day, and increasing the dose to the utmost the stomach can contain and the kidneys can eliminate." Well, maybe not that much, but you get the idea. So drink up!

CHAPTER 10

———

Brain Enhancement and Other
Magical Beliefs

Overall, our knowledge about the human brain remains quite incomplete, and in the gulf of what we have yet to discover lie numerous unanswered questions and unproven theories about various aspects of our experience as emotional, sentient beings. Countless myths have been invented to fill this gulf of ignorance, and among these myths are those concerning normal age-related mental decline and the benefits of herbal remedies purported to restore function in the aging brain. Our brains change throughout our lives, and not always for the better. Why do they change? There are many causes of cognitive decline, including drugs that stimulate GABA receptors too well, calcium channel blockers, dementia and various diseases of the brain and body, head injury, hormone imbalance, dietary nutrient deficiency or excess, heavy-metal toxicity, sleep deprivation, and prolonged stress, to name only a few. The treatments are as varied as the causes. The good news is that sometimes these treatments are relatively effective at assisting the compensation or recovery of a diseased or injured brain.

In contrast, no treatments are currently available that can reverse one of the biggest causes of cognitive decline: normal aging. Put another way, it is impossible to enhance the function of a normal brain as it ages, despite the recent research that has been focused on achieving this goal. This fact has not deterred con artists from placing numerous advertisements on the Internet that claim their products are effective brain boosters or cognition enhancers. In general, these products take advantage of the ability of stimulants to enhance performance. Notice the difference in my terms—stimulants only enhance *performance*, not intelligence or cognitive function. The classic brain stimulants already discussed—coffee, amphetamine, or nicotine—might improve performance, engaging certain neurotransmitters in the process, but they do not raise one's IQ score, and they do not stop normal age-related cognitive decline. The continuing myth of cognitive enhancers relies on the tendency of people to confuse faster performance with real intelligence. We sometimes assume that people who speak quickly are smarter than people who speak slowly. Is there some truth to this assumption? Usually not, but sometimes the answer is yes. Let's take a look at why this might be the case.

One interesting and surprising predictor of intelligence is finger-tapping speed, which is influenced by the level of dopamine in the forebrain. Dopamine plays an important role in controlling the timing of movement. For example, people with Parkinson's disease have reduced levels of dopamine in their forebrain and move slowly. In advanced stages of the disease, these patients also suffer with a slowing of mental function. Research on your brain's timing system, its ticking clock, has often pointed to the important role of dopamine. People who tap their fingers fast usually think fast and their increased processing speed correlates with their IQ score. So how to explain why coffee drinking does not make us smarter? Processing speed for your brain can be compared to processing speed for your computer. Today, most people use computers that process data at gigabytes per second; a few years ago you may have used computers that processed at megabytes per second. We do not assume that the computers are smarter today, just faster. Yet, the way that data can be manipulated makes it appear as though the current computers are better somehow. Your brain is much like this and dopamine seems to be responsible for the clock speed that is tied to your processing speed. More dopamine in the forebrain translates into a faster finger-tapping speed and correlates with a higher IQ than that recorded in people who do not tap as fast.

There are almost certainly many features of your brain other than dopamine release that influence intelligence. Making us faster does not make us smarter. However, drugs that increase dopamine release tend to be stimulants and tend to speed us up and produce arousal; they are also highly abused. There is a good reason why people never use heroin or alcohol to make themselves feel smarter; these drugs do not increase dopamine release in the forebrain. They slow you down and make you act and feel fuzzy-headed and stupid. So why not just take a lot of stimulants and increase your brain's processing speed to the point where you appear to be a genius, even if you're not? The answer is that your brain is probably already functioning almost as fast as is safe. Most of us can push up the processing speed a little without risk. Unfortunately, your neural processing speed in your brain is already just a few extra action potentials per second away from a seizure. Indeed, your brain works so fast that you are always vulnerable to seizures in response to many different stimuli, such as a small head injury, a stroke, rapidly flashing lights, a tumor, vascular abnormalities, or small hemorrhages. Given the limitations of our brain physiology and chemistry, we are probably as smart as we possibly can be at this time in our development as a species.

Your brain is a product of its complex and multi-million year history of solving the problems of survival for its host feeding tube in an ever-changing environment. Some of your brain structures evolved to solve one problem at one point in the evolution of our species and then ended up being used for another, often related, problem. By now, you have seen that the same thing can be said of its neurotransmitters. Overall, your brain is fairly fast but not too efficient, which is probably why stimulants can make us perform some tasks a little better. The brain shows no evidence of being designed in any intelligent manner; it simply works as best as it needs to work to allow us to survive and thrive in our current environment. If that comfortable environment changes sufficiently or too quickly, there is no guarantee that our species will survive. After all, over 95% of all species known to have existed on this planet have already become extinct. No species has had a lock on having a perfect body or brain that allowed it to survive in all environments. The Nobel Prize–winning French biologist François Jacob wrote that "evolution is a tinkerer"—it did not intentionally create anything beyond what was needed at the time for survival. This is why we, and every other species on the planet, are always vulnerable to significant changes in our environment. Overall, the indifferent forces of its environment, not any willful intent, organized your brain. Brain scientists working in this area hold out hope that there might be some wiggle room for improved performance. Thus far, however, no one has been able to design a drug therapy that can make a person smarter in any real way, other than increasing processing speed. So if we look at the so-called memory boosters and cognitive enhancers on the market today, we see that they contain caffeine and sugar and some peculiar amino acids and a few vitamins that together do nothing except make us a little poorer. At this point in time in the 21st century, nothing—let me repeat that—*nothing* exists that can truly make us smarter; so do not waste your money on anything that promises to do so. But do not despair—we can probably age better; some of these solutions are mentioned in the following pages.

Interestingly, some substances that we would not typically consider to be healthy can have beneficial effects on *how* the brain ages. For example, nicotine may be neuroprotective, as may the contents of tobacco smoke, which contains very high levels of chemicals that are efficient chelators of heavy metals. There is, in any case, a reduced incidence of Parkinson's disease among people who smoke. Consumption of large volumes of caffeine-containing drinks is also associated with reduced incidence of Parkinson's disease. The regular consumption of alcohol, primarily beer, has been correlated with a later onset of Alzheimer's disease; this might result from the ability of alcohol to reduce blood levels of cholesterol, which is directly correlated with a greater risk of dementia in later life. Marijuana can be quite beneficial in reducing the onset of age-related diseases that involve brain inflammation, including multiple sclerosis, Parkinson's disease, Alzheimer's disease, Huntington's disease, and a variety of autoimmune diseases. A few recent studies have suggested that people who smoked marijuana in the 1960s are today somewhat less likely to develop Alzheimer's disease.

This is not an advertisement for you to take up smoking cigarettes and pot or drinking beer and coffee because you think doing so will save you from the ravages of these diseases. I mention the beneficial effects of these substances only to emphasize a point: Scientists know about the correlations between the regular use of these popular herbal-based drugs and the reduced incidence of some age-related brain disorders because millions of people have administered billions of doses of these substances during the past thousand years, but only relatively recently has careful record-keeping allowed us to observe the quite subtle, yet very consistent, benefits provided by these drugs. Thus, it is only because these drugs are so widely abused that we've noticed their positive effects on the brain. There may be wonderful new drugs to be discovered in, say, cauliflower or haggis, but too few people have been willing to eat them in sufficient numbers and for a sufficient period of time for epidemiologists to take notice of their hidden benefits on our brain, if they exist.

Many plants do contain compounds that should be able to enhance your brain's performance. For example, potatoes, tomatoes, and eggplants contain solanine and α-chaconine that can enhance the action of acetylcholine. Yet eating these foods does not improve your memory. Your mood should be enhanced slightly by eating fava beans (with or without a fine Chianti) because they contain L-DOPA, a precursor to the production of dopamine, the reward chemical in your brain. The reason that eating fava beans does not make you feel happier is because it is highly unlikely that these ingredients are able to get to their site of potential action at a sufficient concentration that would produce a noticeable effect on brain function. This might explain why no one is hawking potatoes and eggplants as a cure for dementia. But I can assure you that someone somewhere is now selling "*the* cure" for mental decline. I truly wish that a cure did exist; I'd be first in line to get it. We would all prefer to defy the aging process by simply taking a pill and to be able to eat with impunity everything we desire rather than following our mothers' prosaic advice about moderate, healthy eating. But again, and alas, no such cure exists. The fact that science has not yet invented a true brain enhancer has not stopped people from selling drugs, ancient elixirs, unusual therapies with mystical names, and hundreds of books that all boast of the properties of this or that miracle, age-defying brain booster. If someone might gain financially from your gullibility, then what he or she is selling is probably useless, and there is no guarantee that it is safe.

Presently, nothing has been discovered that can significantly enhance cognition or prevent brain aging. In spite of this, people will always be willing to sell you something, be it a book supporting a peculiar diet or a pill containing a special ingredient, which they claim will do so. Why do so many people fall under the spell of charlatans? How can so many people feel so strongly that these drugs work on them? The answer is quite easy to summarize in three little words—the placebo effect. This fascinating effect will be discussed more fully later. Essentially, we want these drugs to do something, anything; so we fool ourselves into thinking that they do. After all, you've just spent a lot of money on this pill! Read on for an example.

GINKGO BILBOA

The Internet is bursting with claims that pills and drinks containing extracts of the *Ginkgo biloba* plant may neutralize free radicals, dilate the blood vessels in your brain, make you smarter, and slow the aging process. How does it do this? The claim is that *Gingko biloba* increases the function of acetylcholine neurons and thereby enhances memory and arouses and improves attentional ability.

Dozens of clinical trials have examined the cognitive effects of gingko plant extracts in humans. A great majority of the studies indicating a positive effect have involved patients who had a mild-to-moderate memory impairment, frequently with a diagnosis of early Alzheimer's disease. Most experiments tested learning and memory, less often, attention. Most of the subjects were selected and tested long after they began using gingko products, typically several months; thus, their cognitive level before using gingko is unknown. This fact may have introduced a bias. For example, higher scores on the memory and learning tests may have come from subjects with better cognitive abilities who could read and understand articles suggesting that gingko might help them or who were better able to remember to take the drug. These critical factors were never considered by the authors of these studies. Testing any drug that claims to enhance cognitive function will have this kind of potential bias in the choice of subjects. At the very least, researchers need to give cognitive function tests both before and after the patients start taking gingko, or else the experimental results showing improved cognitive function from the use of this substance are suspect.

There is another serious problem with clinical trials on plant extracts: determining how much of a given extract a patient should be given, and which extract is the effective one. When ancient Chinese herbalists recommended that their patients take *Ginkgo biloba,* or any number of other plant extracts that have been prescribed during the last two millennia, they always estimated dosage based on past experience. But plants are complicated organisms that make a large variety of molecules, some of which are active in the brain, some of which are not active in the brain but are quite nutritious, and some of which are just inert. Moreover, the contents of plants change according to growing conditions. How much of any particular extract should therefore be taken by a person who seeks the benefit that ginkgo might offer? No one knows! The studies necessary to establish a truly effective dose have never been performed rigorously.

The little research that exists suggests that the ingredients of these herbals have numerous potential mechanisms of action on a variety of neural systems. Unfortunately, there is a lack of unanimity in the research because of various methodological problems in many of these studies, such as inadequate sample size (the number of subjects in the study) and lack of a double-blind, placebo-controlled paradigm, the gold standard of modern scientific research. This paradigm means that no one involved in a drug trial—including its investigators and its subjects—knows which tested substance, whether an active drug or a placebo (usually an inactive form of the drug under study or a sugar pill), is being administered. The purpose of this approach has to do, again, with bias: to keep investigator and subject bias from influencing the trial's results.

In fact, on the rare occasion that this standard has been applied to studies on alternative medicines such as *Gingko biloba,* the results have not been positive. For example, a pair of very large clinical trials that followed the health of more than 3,000 people of various ages for 8 years clearly demonstrated that *Gingko biloba* cannot influence the development of age-related memory problems. Another trial indicated that the use of gingko may actually be harmful, by increasing an individual's risk of nonhemorrhagic stroke, which is when a blood vessel in the brain becomes blocked and shuts off blood flow.

These are, however, just a handful of studies, and much more high-quality research needs to occur before the effectiveness of *Gingko biloba* and other herbal products is irrefutably proven or disproven. In the meantime, most manufacturers of these products prefer to err on the side of selling diluted samples to avoid any toxic side effects and potential lawsuits from people who survive the experience. But that's still no guarantee that the samples are safe. Unacceptably high levels of pesticides and carcinogens have, for example, been found in a large percentage of imported samples.

These concerns aside, many people are convinced that they benefit from substances like *Gingko biloba* or the countless other products on the market that promise enhanced cognitive function. Why? Because, in brief, they want these drugs to do something, anything, so they fool themselves into thinking that they do. We all are subject to this thinking from time to time.

VITAMIN SUPPLEMENTS

Americans spend billions of dollars on multivitamin–mineral supplements, but are they getting a return on their investment? Not always. Numerous studies involving hundreds of thousands of men and women of all ages and genetic backgrounds have found little or no long-lasting benefits from taking a multivitamin–mineral daily supplement. One large study followed the lives of 182,000 men and women; those who took daily multivitamins did not live longer or have less heart disease or cancer, the two primary killers of Americans. In a study following 161,000 postmenopausal women for effects of multivitamin use, those who took daily multivitamins were not less likely to develop breast, ovarian, or any other cancer than women who did not take multivitamins. Among 83,000 middle-aged to elderly men who were followed, those who took daily multivitamins were no less likely to die from coronary heart disease or stroke than were men who did not take multivitamins.

So maybe you're still hoping that taking multivitamins, at the very least, might offer some modest benefits for your substantial investment of time and money. Sadly, after many decades of research, the evidence for even modest health benefits is still very iffy. Even when researchers examined the benefits of multivitamins for symptoms associated with the common cold, they could find no significant health benefits.

What about the brain? Surely, multivitamins help the brain; just look at the hundreds of claims on the Internet! Nope.

When healthy older men and women, aged 60 to 91 years, were given daily multivitamin supplements for 6 months, they demonstrated no significant improvements on memory or other cognitive function tests, as compared to being given a sugar pill. Vitamin E supplements are no longer recommended for brain health; indeed, the high doses originally thought to help slow the onset of dementia with aging are now recognized to increase the risk of cerebral hemorrhage.

In spite of a total lack of evidence that multivitamins offer any real long-term health benefits, we are all addicted to them. This is why Americans are said to produce the most expensive urine in the world; we merely excrete whatever our bodies do not need immediately.

Concerns about vitamins and the balance of their risks versus their benefits were expressed during the early 1950s when parents learned that powerful chemicals—vitamins and minerals—were being added to their child's favorite breakfast cereals. The solution for some manufacturers was to offer the pills as effigies of popular cartoon characters. As recently as 2004, Denmark outlawed some vitamin-fortified cereals because of concerns that extremely high levels of vitamin B6, calcium, folic acid, and iron might achieve toxic levels if eaten daily; the risk is particularly high for young children—the principal consumer of many enriched cereals. The Danes might be overreacting; however it's probably not a good idea to take a daily multivitamin if you're eating a cereal containing 100% of the daily recommended levels.

Overall, most of us are wasting our money because we've been completely sold on the belief that we need these chemicals to be healthy. The epidemiological evidence basically does not support this belief. Indeed, some things that were once thought to be critical for our good health, such as selenium or vitamin A, are simply not as big of a concern; indeed, recent recommendations are to avoid high doses of these two supplements.

However, and this cannot be overstated, some people do need supplements of certain vitamins and minerals, either because of poor diets, disease states, advanced age, gender, or the availability of sunshine, to name just of few of the major reasons. We are all aware of the recommendations that some of us should produce more vitamin D, take folic acid during pregnancy, take certain B vitamins for better mental and physical health, and consume additional iron, particularly if you're a woman over 50 years of age. Given the critical role of iron in brain chemistry, anemia is associated with apathy and depression. Iron deficiency has also been found in children with attention-deficit/hyperactivity disorder. Finally, you should try to get calcium into your diet no matter who you are.

Moderation is still the best approach for most of us: that would include moderation in the number of calories consumed each day, moderation in your daily exercise routine, and a good attempt to obtain your vitamins and minerals from their natural sources. Forget about expensive supplements and just eat small amounts of lots of different foods. Avoid almost anything from

a cow or pig. Obviously, suggesting that you should not purchase expensive dietary supplements goes against everything
you've heard from the people who sell these products. My man-
tra: Save your money and save your brain.

THE PLACEBO EFFECT

When it comes to alternative medicines and therapies that, like
Gingko biloba, claim to enhance your brain function, never underestimate the power of your own expectations. Not only does
your brain influence how you think and feel, but also, by the
nature of your thoughts and expectations, you can influence
how your brain and body functions. Thoughts and brain function form a two-way street; you often feel sad when you are ill
and can think yourself sick when you are depressed. Just like
"The Force" in a Jedi, the placebo effect is strong in some of us
and it can be used for good or evil. One very good example of
the dark side of the placebo effect appeared in the results of a
recent large study of the effects of prayer by large groups of
people on the health of others. When a typical sick person was
not aware that someone was praying for them to get healthy,
their health was unchanged during the duration of the study.
This discovery was in direct contrast to an older, smaller, and
very poorly designed study that widely reported some positive
benefits of prayer. The most interesting outcome of the recent
investigation was that the people who actually were aware that
others were praying for them became significantly sicker. The
authors speculated that the peer pressure to become healthy

produced so much stress that the afflicted patient became even less healthy! I wonder whether we should stop sending get-well cards to people while they're in the hospital. Is that too much pressure on them to get well?

When it comes to alternative medicines and therapies that claim to enhance your brain function, never underestimate the power of your own expectations. Therefore, the best approach, and cheapest one by far, is to expect great things of your brain and generate your own placebo effect. Much has been written about the value of the placebo effect in the practice of medicine, but how this effect emerges and whether it can be controlled are issues that are not yet understood. Essentially, scientists have analyzed the effect based on results of placebo-controlled studies of actual drugs on the brain or have compared only the effects of a placebo against the consequences of no treatment at all. Their findings have been intriguing, if still largely inconclusive. However, in one area of study that is not directly related to an actual treatment, the findings are more definitive. Numerous meta-analyses (which are later analyses of other researchers' data) have shown that only the perception of pain can be statistically demonstrated to be influenced by our minds, which scientists refer to as the emergent property of our brains. This influence of our thoughts and expectations on how we experience pain is a true placebo effect.

In one study, published in late 2008, scientists measured pain perception in two groups of people, devout practicing

Catholics and professed atheists and agnostics, while they viewed an image of the Virgin Mary or the painting of *Lady with an Ermine*, by Leonardo da Vinci. The devout Catholics perceived electrical pulses to their hand as being less painful when they looked at the Virgin Mary than when they looked at the da Vinci work. In contrast, the atheists and agnostics derived no pain relief while viewing either picture. MRI scans demonstrated that the Catholics' pain relief was associated with greatly increased brain activity in their right ventrolateral prefrontal cortex. This brain region is believed to be involved in controlling our emotional response to sensory stimuli, such as pain. Perhaps this study has, in fact, shown us the location of the placebo effect.

Other studies using brain imaging techniques to show correlations between brain activity and the extent of reported placebo effects have demonstrated that some people show greater placebo responses than others, but that everyone appears to be capable of having such a response. There is also increasing proof that the use of placebos might benefit people with Parkinson's disease, depression, and anxiety. In the future, with better testing measures, scientists will likely demonstrate how the placebo effect influences many aspects of our health. In short, the placebo effect is real; we simply do not understand entirely how it works, but the evidence thus far is truly remarkable, particularly with regard to pain. Some people are able to block incoming pain signals or alter how they are perceived. And without a doubt, your mind can make the experience of pain more or less agonizing depending on how you feel—for example, are you fatigued, anxious, fearful, or bored; do you expect more painful experiences to be coming soon?

As noted, your mind also plays a major role in how drugs affect you. Although we don't yet know how the placebo effect works in the brain to influence this process, we do know that it does come into play, and sometimes in surprising ways. For example, the color of the pill you take influences your expectation of what it will do to you. Obviously, pills can be made any color, yet most people like their antianxiety pills to be blue or pink or some other soft, warm color; they prefer their powerful anticancer pills to be red or brightly colored. Americans do not like black or brown pills, in contrast to the preference of people in the United Kingdom or Europe. Thus, almost everything that Americans buy over the counter is a small white, round pill. Yet big pills, or pills with odd shapes, are also assumed to be more powerful, or just simply better, than tiny round pills. Sometimes, a simple change in color or shape restores a drug's ability to produce a placebo effect. And sometimes the effect comes from the pill-taking regimen. For example, you expect that when you are instructed to take a medication only during a full moon, or only every other Thursday, it must be extremely, almost mystically, effective. Herbalists often take advantage of this concept by recommending odd or excessive dosages of peculiar-looking pills or foul-smelling potions. We all want to believe that the pills we take will help us feel and function better; fortunately, thanks to the poorly understood phenomenon of the placebo effect, we do sometimes, but only for a while, benefit even from the most bogus of potions and pills. As Tinker Bell said, "You just have to believe!" If all you're getting is a sugar pill, then does it really matter whether you're fooled into believing the lie? Possibly; it depends on the cost of the sugar pills and the risk one assumes by not taking a medicine of proven effectiveness in a timely fashion for a medical condition. The risk of taking substances that merely promise the elusive Holy Grail of enhanced, age-defying brain function may be no less dire, depending on the true nature of the "sugar" that's in them.

It's so easy to be fooled. Our brains are not as perfect as we would like them to be, and so we keep looking for the magic pill or potion that will make us smarter and prevent the inexorable effects of aging. As long as we keep searching, someone will be there to sell it to us, and we'll stand in line to buy it, none the wiser or healthier and a lot poorer. Still, that does not mean that there is no hope. You have seen that there is one very simple and money-saving thing that we can do to enhance our brain's performance and to slow the aging process: eat a lot less food, because you should never underestimate the power of food on your mind.

FINAL THOUGHT

At the beginning of this book, I stated that my purpose was to demonstrate that we can use our current knowledge of how drugs and nutrients affect the brain to gain a better appreciation of how the brain works. I hope that you've learned that there is a degree of predictability about how your brain responds to drugs and the food you eat. It's not all that mysterious. As you learn more about the brain, whether from the suggested readings I've listed or from other sources, you will become a wiser consumer of both the nutrients and drugs that affect how you think and feel.

SUGGESTED READINGS

Allman, John Morgan. *Evolving Brains.* New York: Scientific American Library, 1999.

Bausell, R. Barker. *Snake Oil Science: The Truth about Complementary and Alternative Medicine.* New York: Oxford University Press, 2007.

Courtright, David T. *Forces of Habit: Drugs and the Making of the Modern World.* Cambridge, MA: Harvard University Press, 2001.

Gold, Paul E., Larry Cahill, & Gary L. Wenk. The lowdown on ginkgo. *Scientific American,* April, 2003.

Lane, Nick. *Power, Sex, Suicide: Mitochondria and the Meaning of Life.* Oxford: Oxford University Press, 2005.

Linden, David. *The Accidental Mind: How Brain Evolution Has Given Us Love, Memory, Dreams, and God.* Cambridge, MA: Harvard University Press, 2007.

Meyer, Jerrold S., & Linda F. Quenzer. *Psychopharmacology: Drugs, Brain and Behavior*, 2nd ed. Sunderland, MA: Sinauer, 2013.

Miller, L.G., & W.J. Murray (Eds.). *Herbal Medicinals: A Clinicians Guide*. New York: Pharmaceutical Products Press, 1998.

Spinella, Marcello. *The Psychopharmacology of Herbal Medicines*. Cambridge, MA: MIT Press, 2001.

Wink, M., & B.-E. van Wyk. *Mind-Altering and Poisonous Plants of the World*. Portland, OR: Timber Press, 2008.

INDEX

ganja, 144
gastrointestinal system, 9, 10, 107, 112,
    182–83
generalized anxiety disorder, 166
genes
    drugs and, 7–8
    obesity, 45
Gingko biloba, 198–201
glia, 11
glucose
    brain function, 32–34
    craving, 18–19
glucose intolerance, 35
glutamate, 153
    age-related changes, 147
    brain development, 155–56
    marijuana, 148
    role in making memories, 161
    turning neurons on, 154–58
glutamate neurons, 23*f*
gluten grains, 179
gluteomorphin, 179
Grant, Ulysses S., 113
Gui Zhi, 57
gut bacteria, balance, 47–48
gut-brain relationship, evolution of,
    9–18
guvacine, 85
guvacoline, 85

hallucinations, *x*, 82–84, 133–34
    barbiturates, 164
    kava kava, 109
    marijuana, 145
    mushroom, 86–87

hallucinogens
    bufotenine, 131–32
    ergot fungus, 130
    LSD, 128–30, 131
    mixing, 139–40
    psilocybin, 130–32
    serotonin neurons, 126–27
Hamlet (Shakespeare), 76, 78
harmala alkaloids, 167
Harper, Bob, 49, 50
hashish, 144
headaches, marijuana for migraine,
    149–50
Helicobacter pylori, 167
hemoglobin, oxygen regulation, 52
hemp, 143
henbane, 75, 76, 78
Henry II (France), 89
Herba Regina, 89
herbe sainte, 89
Hernandez, Francisco, 131
Herodotus, 143
heroin, 18, 22, 44, 102, 110, 111, 175
hippocampus, 13, 23*f*, 66, 67, 138,
    139, 146, 166
Hippocrates, 59, 161
hippy flipping, 139
histamine, dopamine and, 122
histamine neurons, 23*f*
Hitler, Adolf, 101
Hofmann, Albert, 131
holy plant, 89
homeostasis, 66
Homer, 78, 79
hormones